Total Body Toning

Other titles in the
Women's Edge Health Enhancement Guide
series:

Fight Fat
Food Smart
Growing Younger
Herbs That Heal
Natural Remedies

Women's Edge
HEALTH ENHANCEMENT GUIDE™

Total Body Toning

The At-Home Plan for Sculpting the Shape You Want

By Joely Johnson, Gale Maleskey, and the Editors of

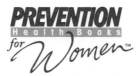

Fitness Consultant: **Jennifer Layne**, a certified strength and conditioning specialist, exercise physiologist, and senior research associate in the Nutrition, Exercise Physiology, and Sarcopenia Laboratory at the Jean Mayer USDA Human Nutrition Research Center on Aging at Tufts University in Boston

RODALE

NOTICE

This book is written to help you make a decision regarding your fitness and exercise program. It is not intended as a substitute for professional fitness and medical advice. As with all exercise programs, you should seek your doctor's approval before you begin.

© 2000 by Rodale Inc.

Illustrations © 2000 by Randy Hamblin, Laura Stutzman, and Tom Ward

Prevention Health Books for Women and *Women's Edge Health Enhancement Guide* are trademarks of Rodale Inc.

Printed in the United States of America on acid-free ∞, recycled paper ♻

Library of Congress Cataloging-in-Publication Data

Johnson, Joely.
    Total body toning : the at-home plan for sculpting the shape you want / by Joely Johnson, Gale Maleskey, and the editors of Prevention Health Books for Women ; fitness consultant, Jennifer Layne.
        p.   cm. — (Women's edge health enhancement guides)
    Includes index.
    ISBN 1–57954–202–6   hardcover
    1. Exercise for women.   2. Physical fitness for women.   3. Women—Health and hygiene.   I. Maleskey, Gale.
II. Prevention Health Books for Women.   III. Title.   IV. Series.
RA778.J599   2000
613.7'045—dc21   99–050050

Distributed to the book trade by St. Martin's Press

  4   6   8   10   9   7   5   3   hardcover

Visit us on the Web at www.rodalebooks.com, or call us toll-free at (800) 848-4735.

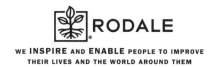

RODALE

WE **INSPIRE** AND **ENABLE** PEOPLE TO IMPROVE
THEIR LIVES AND THE WORLD AROUND THEM

Total Body Toning Staff

EDITOR: E. A. Tremblay
WRITERS: Joely Johnson, Gale Maleskey
CONTRIBUTING WRITERS: Kelly Garrett, Deanna Portz, Julia VanTine
ART DIRECTOR: Darlene Schneck
SERIES ART DIRECTOR: Diane Ness Shaw
SERIES DESIGNER: Lynn N. Gano
INTERIOR DESIGNER: Richard Kershner
COVER DESIGNERS: Lynn N. Gano, Diane Ness Shaw
ILLUSTRATORS: Randy Hamblin, Diane Ness Shaw, Laura Stutzman, Tom Ward
ASSISTANT RESEARCH MANAGER: Shea Zukowski
BOOK PROJECT RESEARCHER: Elizabeth Shimer
EDITORIAL RESEARCHERS: Carol J. Gilmore, Elizabeth B. Price, Staci Ann Sander, Lucille S. Uhlman
COPY EDITOR: Kathryn C. LeSage
PRODUCTION EDITOR: Marilyn Hauptly
LAYOUT DESIGNER: Donna G. Rossi
ASSOCIATE STUDIO MANAGER: Thomas P. Aczel
MANUFACTURING COORDINATORS: Brenda Miller, Jodi Schaffer, Patrick T. Smith

Rodale Healthy Living Books

VICE PRESIDENT AND PUBLISHER: Brian Carnahan
VICE PRESIDENT AND EDITORIAL DIRECTOR: Debora T. Yost
EDITORIAL DIRECTOR: Michael Ward
VICE PRESIDENT AND MARKETING DIRECTOR: Karen Arbegast
PRODUCT MARKETING DIRECTOR: Guy Maake
BOOK MANUFACTURING DIRECTOR: Helen Clogston
MANUFACTURING MANAGERS: Eileen Bauder, Mark Krahforst
RESEARCH MANAGER: Ann Gossy Yermish
COPY MANAGER: Lisa D. Andruscavage
PRODUCTION MANAGER: Robert V. Anderson Jr.
OFFICE MANAGER: Jacqueline Dornblaser
OFFICE STAFF: Suzanne Lynch Holderman, Julie Kehs, Mary Lou Stephen, Catherine E. Strouse

Prevention Health Books for Women Board of Advisors

Contents

Introduction

Women and men. Both have their territory, even at the health club. We women use the treadmills, while men use the weight machines. We do aerobics, they do resistance training. We get thin, they get strong. Isn't that the way it has always been?

Maybe in the last century, but not anymore. Women today can do more than just build stamina and burn calories. We can get firm, strong, and healthy in every way from top to toe! And why shouldn't we? What better way to improve our health and quality of life? So, men, move over. You're going to have to share the equipment. We're getting toned!

But wait a minute. Haven't we done that already? With all those miles racked up on stationary bikes and stairclimbers and rowing machines, haven't we already chiseled ourselves into great shape? You can answer that question yourself. Stand in front of a mirror, hold up your arm, and make a muscle. Firm and toned, top and bottom? Certainly not, if you don't exercise at all. And not if you've done only aerobics because, great as they are for your heart and lungs, aerobics don't make your muscles stronger and firmer. For that, you need resistance training.

Total Body Toning will show you why resistance training is so important to your health and appearance, and it will lead you step-by-step through a makeover so profound that it will actually strengthen your bones! You can pick and choose which muscles to exercise, or you can follow one of four great complete routines. You can do movements that will strengthen you for specific sports, or you can do ballet exercises to improve your poise, balance, and body awareness. You can follow a plan to drop a dress size, get into terrific shape, or maintain your muscle tone. You can even train at the office. And you'll learn exactly how to know whether you are doing your exercises correctly.

Like the other books in the *Women's Edge* series, *Total Body Toning* is full of tips, illustrations, and new information that will help you make use of every advantage that Mother Nature has given us as women, to improve your health in every aspect.

So if you're ready to start being the best you can be, it's time to turn the page. Then, after you've turned through all the pages and spent some time with one of the programs, stand in front of that mirror and make that muscle again. This time, you're sure to like what you see.

Anne Alexander
Editor-in-Chief
Prevention magazine

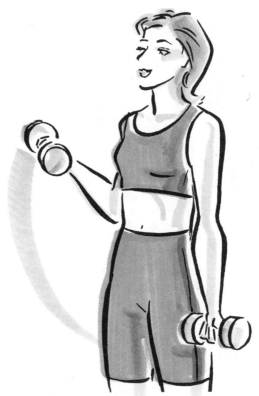

PART ONE

Warming Up to Exercise

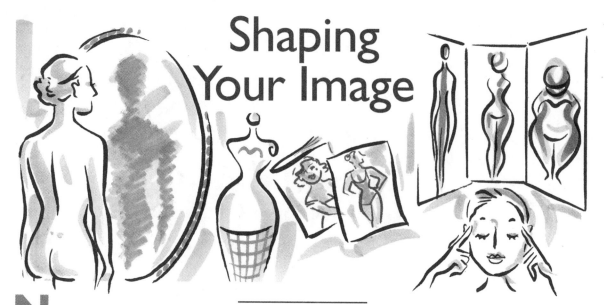

Shaping Your Image

No matter how you look at it—and no matter how it looks—the female body is an absolute marvel. Its design is elegant, its functioning is efficient, and its engineering is powerful. It has the potential to do everything from giving birth to running marathons. In all its shapes, it has inspired artists and poets since the dawn of time, and entire industries are devoted to clothing and pampering it. What a miracle. What a thing to celebrate. How wonderful we are.

Except that many of us have trouble believing in our own wonderfulness.

We look at ourselves, and what do we see? We're too heavy, too lean, too in-between. A national survey shows that more than 40 percent of us are unhappy with some physical trait or another—most often the sizes and shapes of our waists, hips, or thighs. Our body images are terrible, and that can turn even the best of us into wallflowers, sitting out the dance of life.

Think of body image as a 3-D picture of your self-esteem: It's the way you see yourself—for better or for worse—in your mind's eye, ac-cording to Cheri Erdman, Ed.D., professor and counselor at the College of DuPage in Glen Ellyn, Illinois, and author of *Nothing to Lose: A Guide to Sane Living in a Larger Body*. It's a portrait not only of the way your body looks but also of all the emotions—pride, shame, love, or hate—you have for it and how you feel inside of it as you move about your daily life.

Given that our bodies do so much for us—take us through our long lives, give us great pleasures, carry our genetic legacy—you'd think it would be easy to keep a positive attitude toward them, but unfortunately, we don't have control over all the factors that affect the way we think about ourselves. Ever-changing cultural attitudes toward fashion and fitness, as well as men's pref-erences regarding ideal body shape, make up the yardstick that women are given against which to measure themselves.

That's a problem.

When a woman compares her living, breathing body with images she sees in maga-zines, on TV, and in the movies, it's easy for her to feel inadequate and end up disliking her own appearance, says Dr. Erdman. After all, how many of us can realistically hope to look like a fashion model, skinny but muscular, or boylike but busty?

The Lucky Ones

Some of us manage to ignore all the hype and refuse to buy society's line on beauty. In fact, says Dr. Erdman, there are plenty of us, from plus-size to super-thin, who maintain a healthy body image. We are women who love the way we look, the way we move, and the way we feel, regardless of size or shape. Our attitude sets us free. A healthy body image offers other benefits, too.

It eliminates envy. "Being comfortable with yourself makes you comfortable with other women as well," says Dana Schuster, a certified aerobics instructor and cofounder of the Women of Substance Health Spa in Redwood City, California. Knowing how you look and liking it—if not loving it—gives you the freedom to mingle with other women without envy and without cutting yourself down in comparison. We're all different. Diversity is the rule; perfection, the exception. And supermodels are a very rare breed, like snow leopards or bald eagles. They stand out precisely because they are not the norm.

It encourages healthy eating. Eating disorders such as anorexia and bulimia may develop in response to society's demands concerning female appearance. Women

REAL-LIFE SCENARIO
She Doesn't Know When to Quit

Carla has just stepped on the scale for the seventh time today. She doesn't know why, really. She just can't seem to help herself. Every morning, she wakes at 4:00 A.M., runs 5 miles, then goes to her basement to do a free-weight workout, which lasts until 7:30 A.M. Sometimes it goes on longer. Sometimes it goes on so long that she ignores her family and makes herself late for work. Yet in her own eyes, her body still looks undeveloped, so she's working out more and more, and spending more and more time in front of the mirror, examining her shape. She just can't seem to stop. Is there any help for her?

Carla is showing every sign of body dysmorphic disorder, a diagnosable psychiatric condition in which her dissatisfaction with the way she looks is so unyielding that she exercises excessively, rather than healthily. In fact, she may be quite literally addicted to exercise.

So what should Carla do? Her first step is to see a primary-care physician because there are often other underlying conditions—such as an underactive thyroid gland—that lead to dysmorphia. Also, many women with body dysmorphia also have eating disorders such as anorexia or bulimia or both. Or she may simply have given into the intense pressure in our culture to measure up to the idealized bodies we see in magazines and on TV. Ultimately, it's very likely that appropriate psychiatric treatment will help Carla.

As for the rest of us, none of this talk about disorders and compulsions should discourage anybody from exercising with weights. Remember, Carla's case is one of extremes that most of us will never experience. The truth is, a sound strength-training program will help you attain what Carla is missing—healthy self-esteem.

Expert Consulted
Leah J. Dickstein, M.D.
Professor of psychiatry
University of Louisville School of Medicine
Kentucky

THE SHAPE OF PERFECTION

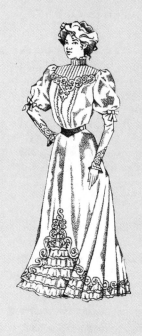

At the end of the nineteenth century and into the beginning of the twentieth century, the standard of female beauty was epitomized by the drawings of Charles Dana Gibson. Illustrations of the so-called Gibson Girls were full of feminine vitality, with a glow of untouched purity about them.

The postwar years of the 1950s brought peace as well as a box-office fixation on breasts. Images of busty stars such as Jayne Mansfield and Marilyn Monroe shaped society's expectations regarding beauty.

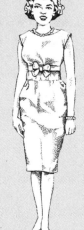

Today's beauty ideal puts the focus on narrow hips, small buttocks, and a taut tummy. Impossibly long, incredibly lean legs are also a sign of the times.

who hold realistic, positive images of themselves are less likely to suffer from these problems. "While bad body image alone is unlikely to propel someone toward an eating disorder, it is certainly a contributing factor," says Sandra Campbell, Psy. D., clinical director of eating disorders services at Brattleboro Retreat in Vermont.

It frees you to get fit. "You can be healthy and fit at any size," says Schuster. Women who know this truth and are accepting of their bodies are free to truly enjoy the entire spectrum of exercise, from dance to weight training. With a positive body image, all options are open and exercise equals everyday enjoyment—not torture to be endured or avoided.

Image Building

It's a Catch-22: If your body image could use a boost, hitting the gym and lifting some weights is a proven way to give it one, says Schuster. But it's hard to work out without shame or embarrassment if your body image isn't positive to begin with.

It doesn't seem fair, but don't throw your hands up and surrender. With time and patience, you can change your mind about your body. It will just take a little creativity and constructive effort.

For starters, try these expert-recommended steps, and work toward appreciating your body the way it is right now.

Apologize to yourself. Entertain the idea that your body talks to you—then listen to what it's saying. Are you hearing love songs or getting hate mail?

It's time to stop the slander, says Dr. Campbell, and even to say you're sorry. Whenever you catch yourself thinking something negative, such as "I'm too fat to lift weights," or "I'll never get in shape," let your caring side intervene. Put a stop to the harmful thought, and apologize to yourself. After all, most women would never speak that discouragingly to others, so why should we say harsh things to ourselves?

Accent the affirmative. Busy women have busy minds. It's time we used that constant stream of internal chatter to do some real good. Affirmations—upbeat phrases that you post in prominent places and repeat silently to yourself whenever possible—are a powerful way to counteract a poor body image. You can come up with your own positive phrase, use a line from a favorite poem or book, or try one of these: "The more I exercise, the better I feel," or "My body is the perfect size for me right now."

Color your world positive. "You need to surround yourself with positive thoughts and positive people," says Schuster.

Step one is to keep your distance from the so-called beauty magazines, which are filled with unrealistic, unattainable images. You won't

WOMEN ASK WHY

It works for Cher, so why won't cosmetic surgery give me any face or shape I want?

Cher looked interesting even before she had any surgery, but many people will give up looking interesting for looking perfectly beautiful in a heartbeat.

While just about anyone can be improved with cosmetic surgery, it's important to realize that the results will vary, depending on where you start. To begin with, each person has her own unique bone structure. This "scaffolding" of the face, as well as the body, is relatively unchangeable. Cosmetic surgery can add height to cheekbones or make your chin a bit smaller, but that's about it. If you are heavy and you also have a large bone structure liposuction can remove the excess fat, but it won't make you small-boned.

Skin thickness also differs, and that can affect the way that certain procedures turn out. For example, a woman with very thick skin may not be as good a candidate for successful nose surgery as a woman with thinner skin.

Generally, it's better to start small than to immediately opt for the most expensive procedure available. If you think you need a facelift, you may actually get great results from having your teeth corrected. A new haircut or color can also make a big difference in appearance. Consult with a qualified board-certified plastic surgeon or cosmetic dermatologist who is willing to discuss both surgical and nonsurgical options before you make any commitments.

If you do opt for cosmetic surgery, remember that the more realistic your expectations are, the more satisfied you'll be with the results.

Besides, do you really want to look just like Cher when you can be you, wonderful you?

Expert Consulted
Rhoda Narins, M.D.
Director of the Dermatologic Surgery and
*   Laser Center*
Manhattan and White Plains
New York

miss out on any groundbreaking news; that's a promise.

The next step, says Schuster, is to choose to spend your time with supportive friends. Find others who are also beginning toning programs, or invite a non-weight-lifting friend to join you in yours.

Exercise Evens the Score

For beating a bad body image, the muscle-building component of physical fitness has much to offer—especially to women. "It's a shame that so many of us overlook strength training, because it can be so much fun and so empowering," Schuster says. In fact, one study showed that resistance exercise betters body image even more than other forms of exercise, such as walking.

Perhaps the most obvious benefit to women is that muscle toning leads to a real—and wonderful—increase in physical power. Movements that were difficult or uncomfortable become fluid and graceful, and actually feel good—making you want to move all the more.

Training with weights also helps women claim emotional power. As our bodies grow stronger, so does our self-esteem. The physical ability to master weights—the ability to literally pull and push them around—naturally results in control over the other facets of our lives.

And, of course, it makes us *look* stronger and healthier.

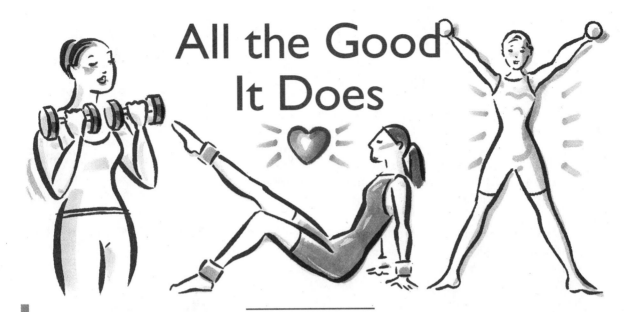

All the Good It Does

If you could have your own personally designed makeover at the world's most exclusive spa, what enhancements would appear on your wish list? You'd want a healthy glow to light your face, of course. And a killer new hairstyle. A firmer body would certainly be a top priority.

But what else? Don't stop there—think big. Imagine a makeover that would give you not only fabulous looks but also extraordinary health.

How about stronger bones, a woman's best friend as time goes by? A healthier heart with better circulation? While you're at it, you may even get a little crazy and throw in a request for a zippier energy level and brighter moods. What do you think?

Well, you asked for it, and you can have it.

Weight training can do all of the above—for cheap, for real, and for good.

A Sculpted Shape

Like the most marvelous makeover imaginable, resistance training fixes flaws from top to toe. Postworkout, your skin will glow naturally,

no cosmetics needed. And after just a month or two, you'll notice improvements that extend where no makeover has gone before—below the neckline.

"There is a definite visual result," says Liz Kelly, Ph.D., professor of physical education and sports psychologist at Monroe Community College in Rochester, New York. "Within 6 weeks or so, there is better muscle definition. This is very motivational stuff."

Women who weight train may see a modest increase in muscle size, called hypertrophy. Hypertrophy is limited by our lack of male hormones. More important, weight-training women will witness an increase in muscle tone, or tonus, which is actually a slight, continuous contraction of your muscles that helps you keep good posture and aids in returning blood to your heart.

As muscles get used regularly through a resistance program, they take on the shape that nature intended. Your biceps, in your upper arms, become smooth on the ends and slightly rounded in the middle. The longer quadriceps, in the tops of your thighs, develop delicious

If, as they claim, lifting weights won't make me too muscular, why do those women bodybuilders look that way?

There are many reasons why professional female bodybuilders look the way they do. First of all, it's possible that they could be using an unusual substance—anything from protein powder or creatine to testosterone or steroids.

Women who take anabolic steroids clearly show muscle hypertrophy (bulking up). The male sex hormone testosterone also has a definite muscle-building effect in women. In one small study of six female bodybuilders who were training for competition, every one proved to be using some sort of vitamin, mineral, or weight-loss aid. While not all athletes supplement their training with such substances, competitive bodybuilders probably have the highest incidence of use.

Some women develop exaggerated musculature simply because they have higher genetic potentials for muscle gain. They naturally have more of a certain type of muscle called fast-twitch muscle, which is easily stimulated to grow by resistance exercises.

Another factor is the amount of time that a professional female bodybuilder puts into building and maintaining her physique. It's really a full-time job. These women are doing tremendous amounts of exercise and eating very restricted diets. Their bodies have extremely low fat content. If you only lift weights for 45 minutes to 1 hour, three times a week, it's highly unlikely that you'll turn out to look anything like a competition-class bodybuilder. It just takes too much work to get into that kind of shape.

Expert Consulted
Janet Walberg-Rankin, Ph.D.
Professor of exercise science in the
*   department of human nutrition, foods, and*
*   exercise*
Virginia Polytechnic Institute and State
*   University*
Blacksburg

definition where the separate bands of muscle meet. And your gluteal mounds in your butt defy gravity and begin to curve voluptuously upward.

Almost unanimously, women react to their firmer flesh with a surge of positive attitude. While we all know that looks aren't everything, an improvement in our curves can inspire confidence and improve self-image. "When you look good, you tend to feel good," says Dr. Kelly.

Better Bones

The gradual loss of bone-mineral density is a fact of life for women as we approach menopause and our previously plentiful estrogen supply diminishes. If our bones continue to weaken as the years pass, osteoporosis—the thinning of bone to the point of dangerous fragility—becomes a real threat to limb and life. Osteoporosis affects more than 22 million American women, and bone fractures due to osteoporosis are heartbreakingly common. Half of all women over 50 will suffer one in their lifetimes.

Although it may be tough to imagine yourself lifting dumbbells at age 80, doing just that may be critical to keeping your bones strong and fracture-free, says Jennifer Layne, certified strength and conditioning specialist, exercise physiologist, and senior research associate in the Nutrition, Exercise

Physiology, and Sarcopenia Laboratory at the Jean Mayer USDA Human Nutrition Research Center on Aging at Tufts University in Boston. The resistance of weight lifting inspires bone to thicken by laying down new layers, especially in spots where muscles attach. Bone density research at Tufts shows that female weight lifters have heavier bone where it counts most—in fragile, fracture-prone places, including the lower back, hips, and wrists.

Bumping up bone density doesn't take much time. Training for just 2 days a week over the course of a year has been shown to enhance bone density of the spine an average of 1 percent, which is a significant amount. Compare that accruement with the expected 2 percent average *loss* of bone density for women who are past menopause and do not weight train.

Weight training also protects bone by improving muscle strength, balance, and coordination, which in turn help to prevent bone-breaking falls.

A Heartier Heart

The changes of menopause can also take a toll on the health of your heart. Lower levels of estrogen put a postmenopausal woman's risk of heart disease right up there with a man's, so you need to take some steps to protect yourself.

Avoiding cigarettes, eating a low-fat diet, and getting enough aerobic

WOMAN TO WOMAN
Standing Up Strong for Her Bones

At 65 years of age, Wanda Archer of Spearman, Texas, is 5 foot 6 and a trim 135 pounds, with a healthy 23 percent body fat. And no wonder she's so fit: She has been a YMCA certified fitness instructor for 22 years. Wanda loves what weights have done for her shape and independence, but recently she's found new reasons to appreciate strength training.

I came around to strength training about 13 years ago when I went to a YMCA exercise seminar that emphasized exercising with weights. I loved the idea of having muscles and being strong. I immediately incorporated strength training into my classes in the small Texas panhandle town where I live. Some of the women weren't too fond of the idea at first. But when they realized what it had done for me, they changed their minds. Strength training has made a big difference in my body shape. I wear sizes 6 and 8 (occasionally a 10). I can carry bags of groceries without strain.

But last year, I was diagnosed with osteoporosis in both hips. Never in my wildest dreams (or nightmares) did I think that would ever happen. I'd been doing everything right since I was 43, when I began regular exercise and taking extra calcium. Exercise was supposed to have made me immune from such a condition.

I was appalled and even angry, but my doctor made me see that my strength training had helped after all. He reminded me that when my sister was my age, three vertebrae in her spine collapsed just because she walked off a small step. Osteoporosis has a strong genetic factor, but nothing like that had happened to me. Strength training had obviously helped.

Something else happened to remind me of the benefits that my strength training brings me. Last year, I tripped over a raised place in a sidewalk, and I could have fallen right onto a flight of concrete stairs. But I was able to catch myself and break my fall, thanks to my muscular legs. Being strong saved me from certain injury that time, and it may again in the future. I know that a lot of women with osteoporosis fall and break their hips, but I'm planning on being too strong for that.

WHAT'S UP WITH THIS?

Creatine

Scan your local supplement shop or grocery store vitamin aisle and step over to the muscle-building bottles. There you're sure to find plenty of products containing creatine, a hot new ingredient that is supposedly "nature's muscle builder." We're talking about popular perception, not claims made by the manufacturer.

Too good to be true? Not necessarily, says Janet Walberg-Rankin, Ph.D., professor of exercise science in the department of human nutrition, foods, and exercise at Virginia Polytechnic Institute and State University in Blacksburg. But some caveats do apply.

Creatine, a combination of three amino acids, is a substance that's normally found in muscle tissue, which means it already exists in your body as well as in any meat that you may consume. In muscles, creatine combines with a substance called phosphate to become fuel for muscle contraction. That's why it can be useful for people who lift weights.

But the creatine/phosphate compound isn't the only fuel that muscles can use. There are others, including fat and glycogen. The body chooses its fuel depending on the demands at hand. Muscles use the creatine/phosphate compound for brief, high-intensity activities like lifting very heavy weights in a hurry, as competitive bodybuilders do. For lower-intensity, longer-duration lifting—like toning exercises—taking in extra creatine probably won't make much of a difference.

Plus, there are some downsides to this supplement, adds Dr. Walberg-Rankin. First of all, not everyone who takes it will see a benefit. "Some seem to respond to it, and some don't." Creatine can also cause rapid weight gain, an effect that most women would probably rather avoid.

More seriously, there's a lack of research looking at the long-term safety of creatine. In one individual case, creatine caused kidney problems. And no one knows what effects the substance may have on pregnant women. "In general, I don't recommend these kinds of things," says Dr. Walberg-Rankin. "It's not really worth any potential risk."

exercise are all proven ways to strengthen your heart and keep your risk of cardiovascular disease to a minimum. Many experts recognize that weight training is another effective way to steer clear of trouble in the heart zone.

When you use your muscles to move weight around—whether it's your own body weight, a hand-held dumbbell, or a stack of weights on a weight machine—the course of blood flowing through your veins is affected. If you are working your legs, your heart directs bloodflow to your lower body to fuel the exertion happening there. Likewise, when you're doing biceps curls, your heart shunts blood to your upper body and arms.

This movement of blood is a good thing, says Layne. Over time, this mild challenge to your heart builds pumping endurance and can help lower your resting heart rate and keep your blood pressure steady. And you can enhance this effect during your workout by alternating upper- and lower-body exercises that encourage bloodflow throughout your entire body.

Energy Forever

If you could make over your metabolism—the rate at which your body uses calories for energy—you'd definitely want to pump up the volume with exercise. As we age and our activity levels lose their spunk, our metabolisms tend to sputter as well. We sit more and exercise less, so our body composition changes for the worse. Without the constant challenge of physical activity, the amount of muscle in our bodies slowly dwindles, while the amount of fat increases. The result is that pounds are gained and energy is drained.

The muscle built through weight training can keep your metabolism on the upswing no matter what your age. That's because muscle is "metabolically active" tissue—it requires a relatively large number of calories to exist. Fat, on the other hand, is metabolically inactive. "Fat just sits there," says Layne. "It's a storage depot."

One study at the Nutrition, Exercise Physiology, and Sarcopenia Laboratory at Tufts showed exactly how muscle boosts metabolism. Twelve older men and women took up a simple weight-training routine for 3 months. They lived at the lab night and day for those 12 weeks, so what they ate, how active they were, and how much they weighed were all strictly monitored. At the end of the study—and with no extra exercise or no dieting—the resistance-training crew needed to eat 15 percent more calories just to stay at their beginning body weight.

That's a substantial spike in how much energy the study participants were generating and the amount of fuel they needed to do it. Fifteen percent is especially impressive when you consider what that translates to in real life. "For an average-size woman eating a 2,000-calorie-per-day diet, that's equivalent to approximately 300 calories, which is an extra small meal or generous snack," says Layne.

So what's the bottom line? Building a

WOMEN ASK WHY

Are isometrics really a waste of time?

When a muscle works against a stationary or immovable object, as when one palm presses against another, the force that's exerted is called isometric. This is in contrast to isotonic exercise, in which muscle force results in movement, as in a leg press or a biceps curl. Isometric exercises have earned a bad reputation as toning tools, but it isn't entirely deserved.

The negative side of working a muscle isometrically is that it won't significantly increase the strength of that muscle. In daily situations, our muscles are usually enlisted to lift, push, or pull, not simply to exert a still force. You *can* generate a lot of force in a static position, but it doesn't translate to real life. Developing isometric strength may therefore be good if you are an arm wrestler, but for normal daily activities, you need dynamic strength—strength that can move an object through space.

Expert Consulted
Jennifer Layne
exercise physiologist
Tufts University
Boston

---

bank of "hungry" muscle mass means that you can eat more calories without gaining weight. If that's not a modern makeover miracle, what is?

Beating Stress and Mending Moods

What makeover would be complete without addressing our innermost form of beauty—our moods and stress levels? Aerobic exercise has long gotten credit for its ability to lift spirits, but you should know that resistance training offers mood-mending benefits as well.

WHAT'S UP WITH THIS?

Steroids

"Steroid," as a word, gets about as much respect these days as "acid rain" or "Saddam Hussein." It's a harmless term for certain kinds of chemical structures. But when you start talking about the anabolic (growth-producing) steroids used by bodybuilders, red flags go up.

Anabolic steroids are essentially synthetic testosterone. The male hormone testosterone is the reason that men who weight train get much bigger muscles than women who weight train. So when you add more of it through artificial means, muscles grow faster than credit-card debt. This leads to the question: Won't anabolic steroids help a woman's strength-training efforts?

They probably will if that woman's goal is to get big instead of toned, says Stella L. Volpe, R.D., Ph.D., assistant professor in the department of nutrition and director of the Center for Nutrition in Sport and Human Performance at the University of Massachusetts in Amherst. They will also help her develop a beard, lower her voice, lose her hair, break out with acne, and treat people with hostility. In other words, the side effects of anabolic steroids are even worse than those that you'd experience if you introduced natural male hormones into your body, says Dr. Volpe.

And there's more. Anabolic steroids have been linked to a higher risk of heart disease, compromised immune system, and manic-depressive episodes, says Dr. Volpe. The bottom line is that anabolic steroids are irrelevant to your toning goals and detrimental to your health.

At least three studies have looked at weight training's potential for relieving depression. In one, 17 people over age 60 who suffer from depression engaged in resistance training twice a week for 10 weeks. Another 15 folks served as a control group—they did no weight training at all. At the end of the study, the group that worked out with weights scored two to three times better on depression tests than the group that didn't lift. "In this study, we see that strength training had as potent an effect as an antidepressant drug," says Layne.

There were also fringe benefits. By the end of the study, the overall levels of body pain among the weight lifters had dropped, and vitality and morale had improved—all of which are especially important in becoming less depressed.

Resistance training also subdues stress—specifically, according to Dr. Kelly, the kind that affects women. "An awful lot of women's anxiety and dependency issues have to do with a feeling of being inadequate in their environments," she says. The strength that is cultivated by a regular weight-lifting routine empowers women, literally and figuratively.

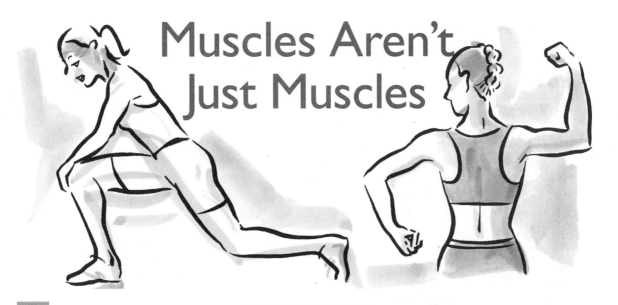

Muscles Aren't Just Muscles

The old saw "In wisdom, there is strength" applies literally to muscles. "The more educated you are about your muscles, the more pleasure you'll get out of exercising them," says Ellen Latham, an exercise physiologist and director of the Eden Roc Resort and Spa in Miami Beach. "Like anything else in life, it helps to have that sense of 'getting it,' of understanding what's going on, and then seeing results."

Making Sense of Your Muscles

Ask any little girl to "make a muscle," and she'll probably flex the biceps on the front of her upper arm. That's a muscle, all right. But so are lots of little tissues throughout your body that keep things moving, from the contraction and expansion of your blood vessels to the moving of food and waste material along your digestive tract.

No trainer has come up with a weight-training routine to work your digestive tract muscles, of course, so your toning task is to exercise only certain types of muscles:

❧ They will be *skeletal*. They get that name for the simple reason that they're attached to bones,

with tough, sinewy structures called tendons doing the connecting. Flex or extend a skeletal muscle, and the tendon will pull on the bone. Next thing you know, you're moving.

Unlike visceral (or smooth) muscles (the ones deep within your body), skeletal muscles are partly visible under your skin, which is why you want them looking good.

❧ They will be *voluntary*. The skeletal muscles you'll be toning move when you want them to move. Not so with involuntary muscles, such as your digestive tract muscles. Nor with your heart. It beats on its own, giving you one less thing in life to remember to do.

❧ They will be primarily *fast-twitch*. Like all body tissue, your muscles are made up of cells. But since muscle cells are long and thin, they're called fibers. There are two basic types of fibers: (1) fast-twitch and (2) slow-twitch.

Fast-twitch fibers are larger, whiter, and, as the name implies, faster to respond to stimulation from the nerves. They're strong and quick because they don't need oxygen to function (in other words, they're anaerobic). These are the fibers you recruit when you do resistance

WOMEN ASK WHY

Why do women have bigger butts and thighs than men?

Since women are in charge of reproductive duties, our bodies reflect that assignment. Our hips are wider for childbearing. We also keep a higher percentage of muscle mass in our lower bodies than men do. But the main reason that our butts and thighs are bigger is because that's where we tend to carry our energy-storing fat.

Not all fat cells are alike. Those in our hips and thighs are better at sucking up available fat, and it's that very fat that provides needed energy during pregnancy and breast-feeding. In fact, during lactation you may notice a reduction of the fat deposits in those parts of your body.

Our tendency to assume a pear shape (as opposed to the apple shape of most men, who tend to carry their fat in their bellies) packs another plus: Fat stored in the thighs and hips is less dangerous than the tummy type because it's less likely to be associated with high cholesterol levels and other cardiovascular problems as well as diabetes.

But there is a downside to this typical female fat pattern, one that you already may have noticed. If you're carrying too much fat on your hips and thighs, it's a lot harder to get rid of it. Remember, you can't target fat loss in any one area of your body, neither through aerobic exercise nor diet. It just doesn't happen, especially in the hip area that gives up its fat so reluctantly.

That's where your toning program comes in. You can't spot-reduce, but you can spot-train. While continuing your overall weight-loss efforts, faithfully perform toning exercises that work the muscles in your fanny and thighs. They'll become firmer and shapelier without shirking their energy-storing duties.

Expert Consulted
Lisa Womack
Associate director of the Cardiac Health and
    Fitness Memorial Gym
University of Virginia
Charlottesville

training, and they're the ones most likely to get bigger and stronger. The downside of fast-twitch? A lack of endurance capacity.

Slow-twitch fibers are smaller, redder, and better at endurance than at strength. They're also highly oxidative, meaning they use oxygen to expend energy. A more familiar adjective describing that process is aerobic.

In chickens, fiber types are all-or-nothing propositions; that's why there's white meat and dark meat. Human muscles, though, are mixed bags. "The proportion of fiber types in each muscle may be 50-50, but it can be as high as 70 percent of one type of fiber," says Priscilla Clarkson, Ph.D., professor and associate dean of the department of exercise science at the University of Massachusetts School of Public Health and Health Sciences in Amherst. "If you have more slow-twitch fibers, you're probably better at endurance. If you have more fast-twitch, you're generally better at sprints."

Your fiber-type proportion is genetic, so it's really true when they say some women are born to be sprinters and others to be long-distance runners. That doesn't mean, however, that you're condemned by your muscle fibers to any one kind of exercise. Women who have a higher percentage of fast-twitch fibers may enjoy strength training more, because they may see results faster, but all women benefit from strength training.

Muscle versus Fat

So muscles are lots of things—skeletal, visceral, voluntary, involuntary, fast-twitch, slow-twitch, and so on. But there's one thing a muscle isn't—a muscle isn't fat.

The difference between muscle and fat is a lot like the difference between a good and not-so-good husband. One is lean and compact, spending a lot of energy to get a lot of things done, and looking good in the process. The other just sits there, saving energy and taking up a lot of space.

Of course, fat cells (unlike husbands) aren't *supposed* to do a lot. "Fat's sole purpose is pretty much to store energy," says Janet Walberg-Rankin, Ph.D., professor of exercise science in the department of human nutrition, foods, and exercise at Virginia Polytechnic Institute and State University in Blacksburg. "Whereas with muscles, there's lots of activity going on all the time. A lot of different processes use up energy."

Women, Men, and Muscles

Truth be told, male and female muscles are pretty much the same. "There doesn't appear to be that much difference in the actual structure of the muscle cell," Dr. Walberg-Rankin says. "No one could look at a muscle biopsy and say whether it's a man's or a woman's."

On the other hand, anybody could look around a co-ed gym and

WOMEN ASK WHY

Why won't lifting weights make my breasts bigger?

When you lift weights, your muscles do the work. It's muscle fiber that's being stressed, and it's muscle fiber that's going to adapt to that stress by growing bigger, stronger, and firmer. Of course, many women would like to add at least one of those three adjectives to our descriptions of our breasts, so why can't we work our breast muscles to make them bigger, stronger, or firmer?

Simply put, there are no breast muscles to work. The human breast consists of fat tissue. So no matter how many bench presses you do, nothing will happen to your breast size. Lifting weights will do a lot of good things, but (thankfully) it won't make your fat cells grow.

Theoretically, your resistance training could *decrease* your breast size, albeit ever so slightly. That's because the increased muscle mass that you develop elsewhere in your body will boost your resting metabolic rate, meaning that you'll burn more calories even when you're not moving. Assuming that you don't eat more to compensate for the difference, your breasts should contribute their share to the resulting fat loss, especially if you complement your toning work with aerobic exercise or a lower-calorie diet. But keep in mind that this is all theoretical. We don't know if exercise actually decreases breast size.

None of this means that weight training has nothing to offer your bustline. On the contrary, exercises to strengthen the muscles under your breasts will improve your chest appearance. Strong, toned chest muscles won't actually enlarge your breasts, but they'll create a healthier and shapelier bust. And that's really what it's all about, isn't it?

Expert Consulted
Priscilla Clarkson, Ph.D.
Professor and associate dean of the department of exercise science
School of Public Health and Health Sciences
University of Massachusetts
Amherst

WOMEN ASK WHY

Why does my husband sweat so much when he exercises, while I hardly perspire at all?

Unless your workouts are very short and very light, sweat is going to join the party when you do your resistance training. Consider it a welcome guest since perspiration is your body's built-in way of thermoregulating—that is, of keeping your body heat under control while you exercise.

There can be lots of reasons why one person will sweat more than another during exercise. But the fact that one person is male and the other isn't probably doesn't have much to do with it, at least not directly. So if you look across the exercise room and see a lot more sweat coming out of your husband than out of you, what's going on?

One explanation may be intensity of effort. He may simply be working harder than you are, expending more energy and generating more heat, and thus requiring more perspiration.

It's also true that highly trained individuals—male or female—sweat more and sooner than their less trained counterparts. There's no inherent reason why your husband should be more trained than you. But if he is, his sweat may be more noticeable. On the other hand, a female athlete who is more trained than he is may outdo him in the sweat department.

Of course, you can also factor in the environment. If you're weight training in your well-ventilated rec room while your husband is working out in a hot, stuffy gym, who is going to sweat more? But again, that's not a male-female thing.

Any or all of these conditions can conspire to extract more perspiration from one person than from another. But since neither toning nor sweating is a competitive sport, it really shouldn't matter. Your body wants to thermoregulate, so it will secrete the amount of sweat that's right for you.

Expert Consulted
Ellen Glickman-Weiss, Ph.D.
Associate professor of exercise physiology
Kent State University
Ohio

see that something is not equal, muscle-wise. That difference is real and permanent, Dr. Walberg-Rankin says, and being aware of it will help you target your toning goals. Male and female muscles part ways in the following areas.

Mass. Most of us accept that men have "more muscles" than we do, but that's a misleading way of phrasing it. Count 'em up, and you'll see it's not true. "What men have is greater muscle *mass* than women," says Alice Ryan, Ph.D., assistant professor at the Veterans Affairs Medical Center of the University of Maryland School of Medicine in Baltimore. "Men are usually bigger and weigh more, so they have more muscle mass in the same way that a heavier woman has more muscle mass than a very thin woman."

That's one of the reasons you see men lifting heavier weights than you'll ever need to.

Distribution. Men pack more of their muscle mass in their upper body than women do. "That explains why strength tests show women much further behind men in exercises involving the upper body than in the lower body," Dr. Walberg-Rankin says. "We're pretty close in leg strength."

That may be a factor if you're planning to compete against men in sports, but not in your toning efforts. "At the elite level, we're still far apart in sports that require a lot of upper-body effort (boxing or lifting) but not so far apart in sports that rely primarily on the lower body (long-distance running)," Dr. Walberg-Rankin says. "If you're working out for general health, though, you should apply a similar effort to all the muscle groups." You'll enjoy the feeling of competence doing lower-body exercises, and the unprecedented strength improvements you'll soon experience in your upper body.

Growth potential. Say you and your husband agree to do resistance training together, using the same routine, the same weights, and the same schedule. Lo and behold, after a month or two, you both notice that his muscles are growing more than yours. What gives? "The difference is that men have testosterone," Dr. Clarkson says. "Without testosterone, muscle fibers aren't going to get much bigger."

That sounds like one more thing to blame on hormones, but it's really a blessing in disguise. Not only should it put to rest any lingering fears you may have about getting "big" or "musclebound" from weight training, but it in no way limits the benefits. "You'll still get stronger, you'll still get improvements in function, and you'll still look better," Dr. Walberg-Rankin says. "You just won't get big like men do."

Why Exercise Tones Your Muscles

By now, you've probably noticed that several terms for the exercises you'll find in this book are used more or less interchangeably: *muscle*

WOMEN ASK WHY

Why is muscle so hard to build when you exercise but so easily turned to fat when you stop?

Your muscles use energy to get stronger and stay that way when your resistance training convinces them that they need to. Stopping your workouts sends them a different message: that there's no need to use so much energy. Being efficient, your muscles quickly revert to their smaller, weaker, flabbier, energy-conserving former state.

But they don't turn to fat, no matter how much the mirror tries to convince you otherwise. A muscle cell can't change into a fat cell or suck up its fat.

Your shrinking muscles' lowered energy demand means that your body is burning fewer calories and perhaps storing them as fat, instead. More visibly, your now-decreased muscle mass—besides being flabbier itself—yields center stage to that persistent fat. And maybe you slacked off on your weight-control efforts at the same time that you stopped your weight training. Muscle doesn't turn to fat, but if you lose muscle and gain fat simultaneously, it may look like that's what is happening.

Muscles shrink faster than they grow for the same reason that it's quicker to tear up a poem than to write one. Muscle building is a complicated biochemical process with lots going on at the cellular level. More important, it's cumulative. You can only make your muscles grow a little at a time by gradually increasing your exercise load.

Unfortunately, body fat works the other way. It isn't "built" like muscles are. It's simply deposited. Eat a thousand calories more than you burn, and those thousand calories settle in as fat right away.

Expert Consulted
Stella L. Volpe, R.D., Ph.D.
Assistant professor in the department of nutrition
Director of the Center for Nutrition in Sport
*   and Human Performance*
University of Massachusetts
Amherst

building, resistance training, weight training, strength training, toning. Read the following summary of how the exercises work, and you'll see why.

If you regularly force your *muscles* to work against *resistance* supplied (usually) by *weights*, they will respond to the stress by building *strength* and improving in *tone*.

Your muscles make this response because they aim to please. "They realize that they're going to be asked to do this task again and again, so they get better at it," Dr. Walberg-Rankin says. "Over time, there's improvement." Physiologists call this adaptation, and it happens in lots of ways.

A matter of nerves. Voluntary muscle contractions are triggered by messages from your brain that are carried through your nervous system. As you can imagine, this is a complicated process, but it functions better with a trained muscle. "Neurological adaptations are the first gains you get from strength training," Dr. Ryan says.

Tapping the force. To repeat, men's muscle fibers are more prone to growth than women's. But what enlargement (or hypertrophy) there is in women should be welcome. "The muscle fibers get bigger because you're packing into them more of the proteins that are involved in contraction," Dr. Walberg-Rankin says. "That means you can generate more force."

Fueling up. Muscles use chemicals like creatine phosphate and glycogen as fuel to perform resistance work. One way they adapt to the demands you're putting on them is to keep their tanks fuller. "Muscles will actually

MEET YOUR MUSCLES

You don't need to memorize the names of all of your muscles in order to tone them. But it helps to be aware of the different areas of your body where muscles are grouped, since you want to work all of them. Here's a look at the most important muscles in each part of your body (and what they're commonly called).

Thighs: Quadriceps, hamstring, adductor, abductor

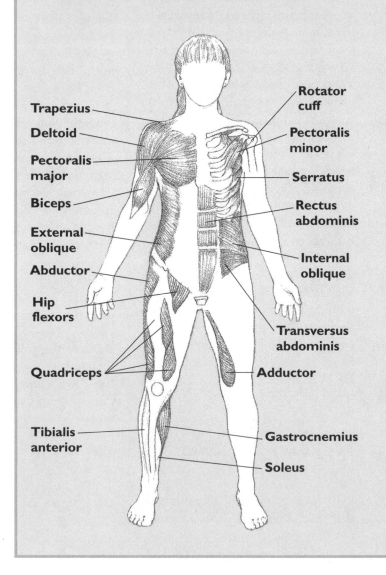

Trapezius
Deltoid
Pectoralis major
Biceps
External oblique
Abductor
Hip flexors
Quadriceps
Tibialis anterior

Rotator cuff
Pectoralis minor
Serratus
Rectus abdominis
Internal oblique
Transversus abdominis
Adductor
Gastrocnemius
Soleus

Calves: Gastrocnemius, soleus, tibialis anterior
Hips and butt: Gluteus maximus, hip flexor
Midsection: Rectus abdominis, external oblique, internal oblique, transversus abdominis
Chest: Pectoralis major, pectoralis minor, serratus
Shoulders: Deltoid, trapezius, rotator cuff
Arms: Biceps, triceps, elbow extensor, elbow flexor
Back: Rhomboid, latissimus dorsi, erector spinae

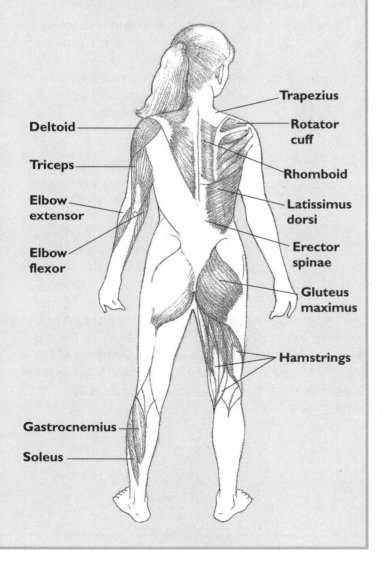

Deltoid

Triceps

Elbow extensor

Elbow flexor

Gastrocnemius

Soleus

Trapezius

Rotator cuff

Rhomboid

Latissimus dorsi

Erector spinae

Gluteus maximus

Hamstrings

store more fuel so they'll have what they need for the next workout," Dr. Walberg-Rankin says. "So the next time you do that workout, it's going to be a little easier for you."

Maximum Adaptation

Your muscles' ability to adapt means they will get toned if you do the exercises in this book. What's more, they *want* to become toned. But you can't just do any old thing and expect results. Instead, keep in mind the following principles of strength training, and watch the improvement happen.

Do enough. You don't need heavy weights, but make sure you use enough resistance so that any movement you do is harder than what you're used to. That's because the whole idea of muscle adaptation is based on the "overload principle," the idea that you have to challenge the muscle into getting stronger. "Doing very light weights isn't going to do much of anything for you," Dr. Walberg-Rankin says.

Keep doing it. If you stop your workouts, you'll lose your tone and strength. Remember, your muscles improved because they were adapting to overload. When there's no more overload to adapt to, your ever-efficient muscles will revert to their previous, less energy-demanding state. "Maintain your workouts if you want to keep the gains," Dr. Walberg-Rankin advises.

Keep moving ahead. Once past the novice stage, the overload principle becomes ever more demanding, at least until you've gone as far as you want to go. For your muscles to adapt, they

POUND FOR POUND, MUSCLE IS BETTER

What weighs more, a pound of muscle or a pound of fat? Okay, you're not falling for that old trick question. But a pound of fat sure takes up a lot more space in your body than a pound of muscle does. That's because muscle is a lean, compact energy consumer, while fat is a bulky, sluggish energy storer. So when you increase your muscle mass with strength training, you're creating a firmer body that will burn fat more efficiently.

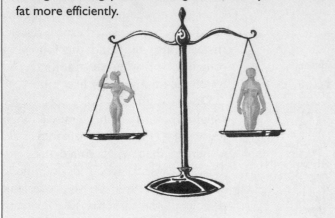

only resistance training is going to get your muscles toned. There's a principle for this: specificity of training. "That's just a way of saying that any improvement is going to be very specific to the type of training you're doing," Dr. Walberg-Rankin says. "Your body is smart enough to only modify those energy systems or muscle fibers that are being called upon."

Work all your muscles. Wouldn't it be great if you could spread the benefits of one weight exercise evenly over all your muscles? Sorry, the specificity principle won't allow it. "You're only going to get improvement in the muscle that's doing the work," Dr. Walberg-Rankin says. "So you have to do a number of different exercises to work all the muscle groups for overall body improvement."

Ease in gradually. Exercising against resistance stresses your muscles. That stress causes damage at the protein level, the repairing of which is part of the adaptation (that is, strengthening) process. Muscle soreness comes from too much stress too soon. "Start off gradually, increase slowly, and you'll avoid most of that unpleasant, sore feeling," Dr. Clarkson says. And if you do get very sore, don't worry. Muscle has a tremendous capacity to repair itself.

need ever-increasing challenges to adapt to. "If you just want to maintain the gains you've already made, that's fine," Dr. Walberg-Rankin says. "But if you want to keep improving, you have to increase the weight or the number of times you lift it or the number of days a week you work out. Something has to keep going up."

Do the right exercise for the job. Other kinds of exercise, such as aerobics, are great, but

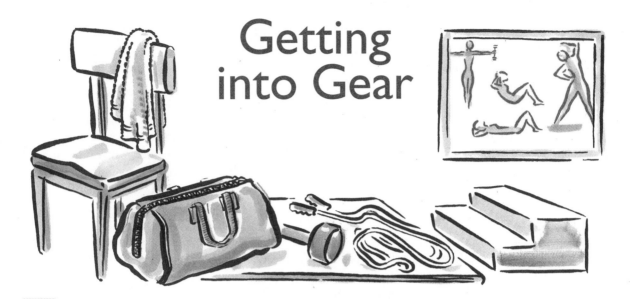

Getting into Gear

Toning up is a personal thing between you and your muscles. You don't need a lot of outside interference from complicated machinery or an array of iron that turns your home into a scrap heap. And you really don't need much space or even a lot of time. All you need is to get yourself ready, mentally and physically.

Getting the gear you'll need is a snap; getting *into* gear can be the hard part. "Women who've never done weight training are probably a little leery about beginning," says Karla A. Kubitz, Ph.D., assistant professor of kinesiology at Towson University in Maryland. "They can feel intimidated because they associate it with studly looking guys in a gym, with sweat flying all over the place. I felt the same way when I started weight training."

So there you have it. If even exercise professionals have to overcome mental barriers to start their resistance-training programs, you're in good company. But these are barriers that are made to fall. Once they do, you'll be surprised at how easily the more mundane issues of time, space, equipment, and clothing will come together for you.

Break On Through

Resistance to resistance training is so common among women that breaking through the mental barriers has become a subject of behavioral psychology. We go through stages before we're ready for any new behavior pattern, be it quitting smoking, changing our diets, or toning our bodies. If the idea of starting a weight-training program seems daunting to you, it's not because you're weak or lazy. You just haven't moved through the stages yet.

Take a look at the following thumbnail sketch of typical behavior-change stages, and see where you fit in.

Stage 1: Pre-contemplation.
You think: "Weight training is useless, and I don't even want to hear about it."

You need: To read this book.

Stage 2: Contemplation.
You think: "Maybe there's something to this weight-training thing after all."

You need: To weigh what you will put in to a muscle-toning program against what you will get out of it.

Stage 3: Preparation.

You think: "I'm sold, so what do I do?"

You need: Practical knowledge to put your readiness into action.

Stage 4: Action.

You think: "Hey, I'm really doing it!"

You need: To see some results.

Stage 5: Maintenance.

You think: "Weight training is now part of my life."

You need: Support strategies to keep it that way.

Simply being aware that these stages exist is helpful, Dr. Kubitz says. "You can see that you're actually getting somewhere just by thinking about weight training, even if you haven't actually done anything. Just going from pre-contemplation to contemplation is progress." But there's more. When you know where you stand, it's easier to take advantage of some of the barrier-busting ideas that experts offer.

Do your legwork. There's no surer formula for failure than to hit the weights willy-nilly. "You can't take a contemplator or pre-contemplator and just stick her into an exercise program," notes Dr. Kubitz. "She's not going to benefit because she's not ready for it."

How do you get ready? By getting smart about the benefits of resistance training, the equipment you'll use, the exercises you should do, and the way you should do them. "Do your research before you do anything else," says Vicki Pierson, a certified personal trainer at the Fitness Jumpsite in Chatanooga, Tennessee.

Talk to yourself. "I just can't do it." Sound familiar? If you've convinced yourself that weight training is beyond your capacity, convince yourself otherwise—out loud. Verbal persuasion, as it's called in theoretical circles, helps break that confidence barrier. Encouraging words from a trusted friend will work wonders, but if no such friendly words are forthcoming, do the talking yourself. "You can provide your own verbal persuasion," Dr. Kubitz says. "Start telling yourself that you *can* do it."

Seek a role model. Seeing is believing, and there's nothing more inspiring than seeing someone who is no different from you tone up successfully. "Find somebody who's done it and who's just like you in terms of sex, age, and other characteristics," Dr. Kubitz says. "Then you're more likely to think that you can do it, too."

Another source of this "vicarious experience" (the behavior-theory term) is your own mind. "Just start imagining yourself doing it," Dr. Kubitz suggests.

Stack the deck. Previous experience at something boosts what researchers call your self-efficacy—that is, your belief that you really can do this thing. The applicable cliché is "Success breeds success." But if you're a beginner, by definition, you haven't had any success to breed with. Your course, then, is clear: Cheat.

Well, don't *cheat*, exactly, but rather rig the game in your favor. "Start your weight-training program with something you're sure to succeed in, something designed to work," Dr. Kubitz advises. That means setting easily attainable goals at the outset. Modest as they may be, achieving these little goals gives you success to build on and sets the positive cycle spinning.

"After just a few weeks, you define yourself in different ways," says LaJean Lawson, Ph.D., adjunct professor of exercise science at Oregon State University in Boring. "You start thinking, 'Hey, I feel like I know what I'm doing here.'"

Relax. Do you more often picture yourself klutzily dropping a weight on your toe than triumphantly lifting it into the air? Do you think you're more likely to look silly in the short run than toned in the long run? Beginner's nerves are to blame, and they're a common barrier when it comes to working with weights. "If you get really nervous just thinking about this thing, you're less likely to start doing it," Dr. Kubitz says.

Dr. Kubitz recommends basic relaxation techniques to overcome this particular obstacle. "It's not really complicated," she says. "If you can just take some deep breaths before you do anything, you can change your physiological state. Relax, think positively, and imagine yourself feeling okay while you're doing it. Then go and do it."

Deal with those barriers. It's funny how practical problems like finding the time or the space in which to do your toning exercises can become insurmountable for those still in the contemplation or preparation stages. Don't let that happen, says time-management consultant Virginia Bass, owner of By Design, a personal and professional development company in Exton, Pennsylvania. "Make a written list of what your barriers are and come up with solutions for them. Negotiate your barriers before they turn into problems."

Tone at home. Working out at home may be the best way for some self-conscious women to start, says Sandra Campbell, Psy. D., clinical director of eating disorders services at Brattleboro Retreat in Vermont. You can make great strides with simple equipment: Team a pair of inexpensive handheld weights with a variety of toning videos, or use them with your own resistance-workout routine that you've written down in advance.

WHAT'S UP WITH THIS

Sauna Belts

Remember the portly young gentleman in *The Full Monty* who wrapped plastic around his midsection in the hope of losing weight in time for his striptease performance? Sauna belts are a variation on that theme—and just as useless for toning up or trimming down.

Toning is about muscle cells. Weight loss is about fat cells. But sauna belts are about water. You wrap one around your midriff to sweat away inches as you work out. "It's the same idea that wrestlers use when they put on those plastic suits to sweat themselves down to their weight class," says LaJean Lawson, Ph.D., adjunct professor of exercise science at Oregon State University in Boring. "Sauna belts cover just the midsection, but the full-body versions, like rubber or plastic suits, are actually dangerous. You can make yourself dehydrated."

With so many health and appearance benefits to be gained from anaerobic and aerobic exercise, sauna belts are, at best, a distraction. Still, lots of them are sold to women, perhaps because they "work" in the sense that the tape measure may show a smaller number after you wear one. That number reflects nothing but a temporary water loss, which is hardly what you want. "It's totally bogus," Dr. Lawson says.

Find a user-friendly gym. When you are ready to take the public plunge, consider your options carefully. Some health clubs seem to be overflowing with perfect specimens. These are the places that are likely to double as social clubs for singles on the hunt. If that sort of atmosphere makes you uncomfortable (and, really, how could it not?), look for a gym that's a little more down-to-earth, says Dr. Campbell. There may even be a place that caters specifically to your needs. Check out women-only gyms, like some Lucille Roberts locations, or size-friendly facilities, like the Women of Substance Health Spa in Red-

HOOPING IT UP

Maybe we were onto something when we whittled away all those hours of our childhoods playing with hula hoops. Now we can use the best thing that ever came out of the 1950s to help whittle away at our waists. Hula hooping is fun proof that just about anything that gets you moving can get you healthier—and it can help tone your midsection, too. But you have to use it right to get the benefits, says Vicki Pierson, a certified personal trainer at the Fitness Jumpsite in Chattanooga, Tennessee. So remember these three tips to help keep that hoop moving.

1. Keep your abdominals contracted as you twirl the hoop.
2. Keep your back straight while moving your hips around in a small circle. Don't sway from side to side.
3. Keep it up until you really start feeling it in your abdominals—and then keep it up a little longer.

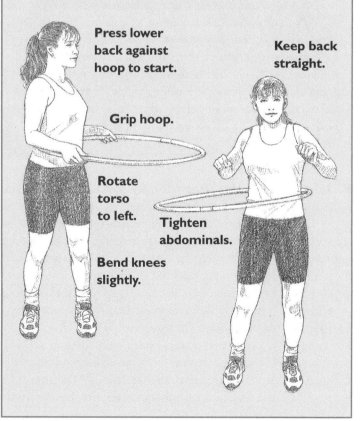

Press lower back against hoop to start.

Grip hoop.

Rotate torso to left.

Bend knees slightly.

Keep back straight.

Tighten abdominals.

wood City, California. If that's not an option where you live, don't lose heart. Instead, try to visit a more generic gym during its least crowded hours. With fewer bodies bustling for places on benches or seats at weight machines, you'll find the atmosphere a lot less intimidating. Another plus: When you ask for pointers from the staff, you'll have their undivided attention.

The Right Stuff

With so much fitness equipment out there, it's easy to assume that muscle toning requires a major capital investment and a schedule overhaul. It doesn't. The truth is, your needs pretty much come down to a few simple weights to lift, a little bit of time to lift them, and somewhere to do it. What matters isn't getting the most stuff—or the most costly stuff—but getting the *right* stuff. And that turns out to be not much stuff at all.

You'll be pleased to know that time requirements are nice and flexible when it comes to body toning. All that matters is that you're consistent. "You accomplish your goals by completing exercise tasks over and over on a regular basis," says Ellen Latham, an exercise physiologist and director of the Eden Roc Resort and Spa in Miami Beach. "Success comes from doing it regularly."

Doing it regularly is not the same as doing it a lot. "You don't have to spend a great deal of time to get the benefits," says Karen Snowden Rucker, M.D., editor in chief of the

Journal of Back and Musculoskeletal Rehabilitation in Richmond, Virginia. "It's much more important to do what you can maintain than to try to push things."

Take your time. You need to pick a time of day to work out, experts say. But they're not saying when that may be. "Physiologically, there's no best time to do your workout," Latham says. "The best time is the time when you're going to do it. It's up to you to look inside yourself and decide when that is."

So it's your call, but you may want to try mornings first. "I find that a lot of people have success doing their exercise first thing in the morning, before the kids are up and before they have to get ready for work," Latham says. "Once their day starts rolling, they're too busy."

Keep that appointment. Once you decide on a time, don't write it in your agenda—write it in stone. A firm, must-do exercise time is essential for success. "You have to have it set in your mind that this is an appointment, something you can't not do," Latham says. But, you protest, if it doesn't matter what time of day you work with weights, why can't you just fit it in when you have time to kill? "Because it won't happen," Latham insists. "Something else will take precedence. You have to make an appointment with yourself."

Do your make-up work. Sacred as your set time may be, missing it doesn't have to mean missing your workout. Tap your creativity, and you'll find the make-up time. "If you're just sitting there watching television, you can get up and do the weights then," Dr. Rucker says. "Working out right before bed will probably interfere with sleep, so leave about an hour of down time after your workout before you catch your Zzzs."

Lunch hour is another possibility. "You want to give adequate time for digestion, but it's not like the old theory that you have to wait at least an hour before jumping in the pool," Latham says. "Just wait long enough so you're comfortable with the movements that exercise requires."

A (Weight) Room of Your Own

All of the exercises in this book can be done in your home with no fuss and no muss. The equipment you need can fit in your closet, so it doesn't matter if you live in a studio apartment with four kids, two dogs, and a hamster, or by yourself in a mansion. Any place is suitable for temporary conversion to a workout space, Latham says, as long as it meets the following three requirements.

1. It's safe. That means that there is enough room to do the movements without damaging your precious belongings or your even more precious body. "Go ahead and clear a space in your living room temporarily, if that's your only option. Just make sure you really clear it. You don't want to be banging into coffee tables."

2. It's relatively private. You don't have to hide while you work with weights, but you do want to concentrate. "Try to find an area where you can focus on what you're doing—a side room or a bedroom, if that's possible. If you're right in the middle of traffic, with kids running in and out, you won't be able to give the work the dedication it needs."

3. It's ventilated. Shutting out the kids and the cold are worthy goals, but don't suffocate in the process. "You're going to be increasing your body temperature, so you definitely want some air circulation going on wherever you're doing the exercise."

The Right Tools for the Job

Some people fill their bookshelves with books that they'll never read. It's easy to make the same mistake with home toning equipment. Better to concentrate on the basics and add the little extras later. Here's what you'll need.

Dumbbells. These are the mainstays of your resistance-training program, the actual "weights" that you'll be "lifting" for most of the exercises. You grip a dumbbell, usually with one hand, around the cylindrical middle. Most of the weight is on a "head" at either end.

In a weight room, the heads are removable plates that range from the size of a compact disc to the size of a pizza pan. Don't even consider getting a set of those, Latham advises. "Most women prefer the dumbbells with smaller heads that are more like knobs at the ends," she says. "The movement is smoother, and they're easier to manipulate." Each will have a set weight, so it's a good idea to start with six dumbbells—three different weights for each hand. If you're a beginner, that may be 3, 5, and 7 pounds, with 10 pounds probably the upper limit. You can get heavier dumbbells as you get stronger.

Ankle weights. You can do some lower-body exercises by using handheld weights while lunging, stepping, or squatting. Others, though, require some weight right where the action is. So unless you can grip dumbbells with your toes (please don't try), you're going to need some ankle weights to work your southerly muscles. An ankle weight is nothing more than a piece of weighted material that you wrap around each ankle. Your best bet is to get the kind with pockets or sleeves into which you place little bars to adjust the weight. That way, you don't have to buy more than one pair, and you don't have to

take the darn things on and off during your workout.

A step bench. This can be the same kind of strong plastic bench used in aerobics classes. This type is sturdy but light, and it will help you work your calf muscles, among other things.

A full-length mirror. This may sound like a luxury option, but it's obligatory. Vanity is not the issue; self-observation is. "Form and technique are everything," Latham says. "A mirror is important for making sure that they're consistently correct."

An exercise mat. Both you and your dumbbells are going to be spending some workout

After 3 years of frustration, I decided that I wanted to be fit and healthy as well as to lose weight. I admired other people who were that way, so why couldn't I be, too? When I started fitting an exercise program into my schedule, I finally began to see some lasting results. After 6 months of weight-training and aerobic workouts, I've lost 15 pounds (with 25 still to go).

I'm also starting to see some muscle definition from the strength training. And I love the way it makes me feel so strong.

Time hasn't been a problem, even though I do my aerobic work five or even six times a week, and I work with weights three times a week. I usually exercise before I go to work and sometimes when I get home. For aerobics, I use videos, and I also take a 40-minute walk about once a week. For strength training, I have a variety of dumbbells, from 3 to 20 pounds, as well as a barbell and a bodybar (a heavy, vinyl-clad bar that you lift like a barbell).

It's all very simple. I exercise at my own level, not somebody else's. And since I found something that I love to do, it doesn't seem like I'm spending a lot of time with it. Compared to the 3 years that I spent with no results, exercise is as time-efficient as you can get.

time on the floor. You need a mat for comfort and to protect your floor surface. For durability, you should look for a mat with 1-inch-thick polyethylene foam that is not too firm and not too squishy.

A sturdy chair. You do some exercises while sitting down. For a toning program, a sturdy, high-backed but armless chair—a dining room chair, for example—will do just fine.

An exercise bench (optional). You may prefer a small, padded exercise bench to raiding your dining room for a sturdy chair. It makes more positions possible—especially prone ones—and will fit nicely in your closet when not in use.

Gloves (optional). Hard-core lifters sometimes wear gloves to protect their hands from calluses as they move large quantities of iron around. You don't need them, although some women feel more comfortable when they wear gloves to improve their grip. If you're one of them, use gloves that are made for resistance training, not your snow mittens.

That's it. Hardly a checkbook-challenging shopping list, is it? And everything is easily findable. In fact, the only complicated thing about buying basic resistance-training equipment is sorting through the huge selection available. Here are some ways to simplify the task:

Buy live and in person. Not all personal exercise equipment that is offered through television shopping channels and the Internet is bad, Latham says, but it's not the best way to outfit your little home gym. "There's just no way to know for sure what you're getting," she says. Instead, she advises, check out your choices firsthand at sporting goods stores or other retail stores that stock fitness equipment.

Test-drive. Even if it's brand new, anything that you buy should be used—by you, right there in the store. Pick up lots of dumbbells and find a grip size that fits your hand and a feel that you like (there are several choices of material, including plastic coating or chrome). Walk around in ankle weights, sit on benches, step on steps. "Try the equipment on like a pair of shoes," Latham advises. "Use it; feel it; do everything but taste it."

Kick the tire. Besides personal preference, check for quality. How can you judge? "It's really simple: If something feels flimsy or cheap, it is," Latham says. "You can tell if that dumbbell is awkward or that bench is shaky. You just need to pay attention."

Dressed to Tone

The best weight-training outfit is one that you're unaware you have on, Dr. Lawson says. The last thing you want when you're working your muscles is a stifling sleeve, a wayward strap, or shoes that hurt. "First and foremost is comfort."

But image counts, too. After all, we're talking about clothes here. "With resistance training, there's an emotional process of putting yourself in a new role," Dr. Lawson adds. "When you wear the right clothes for exercise—a sports bra, for example—you're identifying yourself as an active person."

Let it show. Wear clothes that expose your arms and legs. Not only will that help you maintain proper form, but it will also give you a better view of your progress. "Assuming that you're not working out in a cold place, shorts and a tank top or T-shirt are great to work out in," Dr. Lawson says. "You want to see your muscles working and starting to emerge. Women tend to carry less fat in their upper bodies, so the results can be seen there fairly quickly."

Commit a strategic cover-up. Being comfortable also means not feeling self-conscious. "If you're really body conscious, go ahead and keep that T-shirt loose if your midsection isn't what you want it to be right now," Dr. Lawson says.

Try bike shorts. Spandex bike shorts are popular for good reason, according to Dr. Lawson. They're form-fitting so you can see the muscle action in your upper legs; but at the same time, they're nice and light. "Those stretchy fabrics are just so comfortable," Dr. Lawson says. "And women like bike shorts because they act like an exercise girdle, making us look firmer the moment we put them on. Get bike shorts with Power Lycra in them, and they'll help you firm up in a big hurry." They're made with high-stretch and high-compression fabric that reduces muscle vibration—the major cause of fatigue.

Cross your shoes. Dr. Lawson recommends using shoes that are sold as cross-trainers. "You'll get the support and traction you need, so you won't be slipping around with the weights. But you can also do your walking, jogging, or biking without switching shoes."

Don a sports bra. For working with weights, the support and breast-motion control that sports bras are known for tell only part of the story. Unlike its everyday cousin, a good sports bra will stretch effortlessly and from the back, allowing you easier movement. Its straps won't press on your shoulder muscles or (worse) fall down while you're moving dumbbells around. And its fabric is designed to wick away moisture from your skin. "The whole point is to get your mind off your bra and onto your workout," Dr. Lawson says.

Pleasure, Not Drudgery

"You'll stay with it if you enjoy it," Latham says of resistance training. The trick is to put pleasure into your toning routine without losing concentration. Watching *Jeopardy* while you do your 30 minutes on an exercise bike is fine, but when you work with weights, it's best to add elements that will help you focus, rather than distract you.

Turn on the music. "Music is a wonderful source of exercise motivation," Latham says. That observation is supported by research, clinical practice, and millions of panting aerobics enthusiasts. But music is also a treasure of pleasure for your weight routine. Music works its magic in a myriad of ways, according to Cheryl Dileo, Ph.D., professor of music therapy in the Esther Boyer College of Music at Temple University in Philadelphia and past president of the World Federation of Music Therapy and the National Association for Music Therapy. It will improve your mood, help structure your movements, fend off fatigue, combat pain by stimulating the production of endorphins (natural feel-good chemicals), reduce tension, enhance concentration and focus, and make the time fly by faster. (Too bad it doesn't lift the weights for you, too.)

Be a good deejay. Another advantage to home workouts is that you can pick your own music. And that matters, Dr. Dileo says. "Select music that you enjoy and associate with positive memories or experiences. You may select music with lyrics that affirm what you're doing as your exercising. Sing along with the lyrics if possible, even if only in your mind."

Dr. Dileo also suggests that you use music with a pulse that matches your workout. "Move and breathe to the music to structure movements and prevent fatigue," she says. "And feel free to change the music often to prevent boredom." The tempo of the music should match the tempo

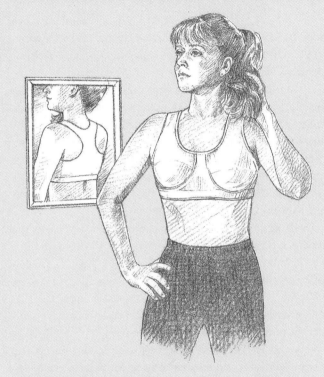

A Sports Bra Works Wonders

A good sports bra has a lot more to offer your toning workouts than support and motion control (although you'll get those, too, of course). Here's what to look for.

A higher neckline: Not for modesty, but to prevent riding up

Moisture-transport fabric: To wick away sweat

Nonabrasive fabric: No rough stitching, threads, or seams

Cushioned or plastic underwire: To feel secure, not poked

A wider rib-band: To keep the bra anchored

Stretch in the back: For easy arm and body motion

No metal against skin: Hooks, if any, cushioned in fabric

Broad shoulder straps with a Y back: No falling down, no undue pressure

WOMEN ASK WHY

Why do women always inherit their mothers' thighs, not their fathers'?

The fact that women tend to store more fat in their hips, buttocks, and thighs has more to do with biology and hormones than genetics. In other words, it's a female thing.

Women are typically pear-shaped because of the way an enzyme, lipoprotein lipase (LPL), acts in certain parts of their bodies. LPL removes triglycerides (fat) from the blood and puts them into the fat cells for storage. In women, there's greater activity of this enzyme in the thighs and butt, so these areas are the most efficient at storing fat.

In men, LPL is most active in the abdomen, which is why guys tend to pack extra pounds around the middle.

The female hormone estrogen is probably what directs the enzyme's activity to be greater in the thighs and butt. Women's bodies are designed to tap into those fat stores during pregnancy and breastfeeding.

Women also have more room to store fat under the skin in an area called the subcutaneous fat layer. That layer is 8 percent thicker in women than it is in men.

So when it comes to your thighs and rear, here's the bottom line: Don't blame your mother for your larger lower half—blame Mother Nature.

Expert Consulted
Michele Trankina, Ph.D.
Professor of biological sciences and nutritional
*   consultant*
St. Mary's University
San Antonio

of your particular routine. If the routine is done nonrhythmically, it may be better to choose music without a particular, structured rhythm, such as new age music, she says.

Look good. Anything is more fun when you look good doing it, right? That fact of life applies to resistance training, too, according to Bass. "A nice outfit that's colorful as well as comfortable is going to be stimulating," she says.

If it feels good, do it. Working with weights is not supposed to feel bad. "A lot of times, women try to do an exercise that doesn't feel good and think that it's not supposed to," Dr. Rucker says. "But a movement shouldn't feel awkward. If it does, you may be using too much weight or be in the wrong position."

Keep your eyes on the prize. Visualize in your mind's eye the "you" that you're doing all of this for, suggests Latham. "See yourself looking great in that swimming suit. Or see yourself as an energized person with a skip in her step at the end of the day, instead of someone who is slumped over and broken down. Keep picturing why you're doing what you're doing, while you're doing it."

Part Two

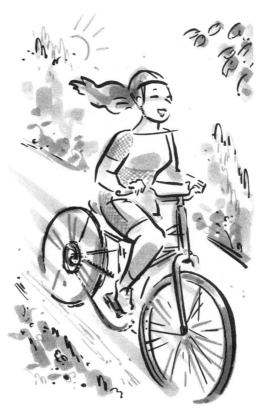

Muscles
in Motion

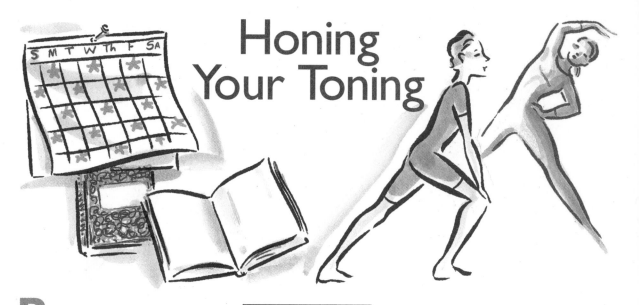

Honing Your Toning

Be prepared. That's the Girl Scout motto. And it's as true for starting a toning program as for anything else.

Resistance training isn't simply picking up a dumbbell and putting it down. There are aspects of the art of toning that make working out, especially with weights, safer, more effective, and more fun. Even if you're so eager to pump some iron that your triceps are twitching in anticipation (all right, so maybe you're not *that* eager), first take a moment to learn to do it the right way.

Go for a Goal

Before you begin using the exercise program that follows, you need to decide on a goal. Each exercise is presented with three options: Drop a Dress Size, Shape Up, and Maintain. The options are slightly different when it comes to the amount of weight you'll be lifting and the number of repetitions you should do.

To choose the goal that's right for you, look over the following descriptions.

Drop a Dress Size. If you're primarily interested in firming up spots that jiggle, this is the category to choose. But remember, although these exercises may help you reduce your size by toning and tightening your muscles, they won't make you lose weight.

Shape Up. If you're satisfied with your present size but would like to see more definition and feel more strength in your muscles, follow these directions. This exercise category will challenge your muscles and help to carve out the sexy shape that you crave.

Maintain. You're already right where you want to be. Possibly through weight training, you've reached the size and shape of your dreams. Lucky you! Your job now is to maintain the gains you've made, by adding variety to your program and staying motivated. You'll be able to do just that by using the directions in this category.

When it comes to selecting the proper amount of weight to lift, always begin with the lowest weight recommended for your range, according to Jennifer Layne, certified strength and conditioning specialist, exercise physiologist, and senior research associate in the Nutrition, Exercise Physiology, and Sarcopenia Laboratory at the Jean Mayer USDA Human Nutrition Research Center on Aging at Tufts University in Boston. Perform one set and see how long it takes you to feel ready for a second set. You should need to rest for at least 30 seconds and no more than 2 minutes between sets. If you need more than 2 minutes to gear up for the next round, the weight you're lifting is too heavy. Choose a lighter load for the next set. Also, if you have no delayed-onset muscle soreness after 24 to 48 hours, you have the green light to increase the amount of weight incrementally.

Turn Up the Heat

You preheat the oven before sliding the brownies in. In winter, you let the car idle for a moment or two before putting it in gear and zooming down the road. You should also warm up your muscles before resistance training.

Muscles that are "cold" are less flexible and actually shorter. When you ask a cold muscle to get longer in a hurry by picking up a weight, you run the risk of pulling or even tearing that muscle. Warming up gradually lengthens a muscle and sends more bloodflow to the area, which dramatically reduces your chances of injury. A proper period of warming up also helps to get you up to speed mentally. Taking a few minutes to prepare for your toning session al-

WOMEN ASK WHY

Why has the number on my scale been going up since I've been going to the gym, while my dress size has been going down?

If you are just starting out with a resistance-training program, your weight actually shouldn't fluctuate too much. A couple of pounds' change either way is normal, depending on whether you ate or drank before stepping on the scale, and, to be honest, the time you last used the bathroom.

If you've gained more than a couple of pounds but your body is shrinking and getting firmer, don't worry about the weight. It's your underlying body composition—the amount of fat versus the amount of muscle—that matters more than the number on the scale. Here's why.

When you weight train, you are working on increasing the amount of muscle in your body and decreasing the amount of fat. Pound for pound, muscle takes up about 22 percent less space than fat. Think of it this way: If you could put a pound of muscle and a pound of fat next to each other on a table, the muscle mound would be about three-quarters the size of the fat mound, even though they weigh the same.

Rather than focus on your weight, you should pay attention to your clothing size. While some women will drop pounds through resistance training, weight loss is a different goal from the aim of becoming stronger and more toned.

Expert Consulted
Jennifer Layne
Exercise physiologist
Tufts University
Boston

lows you to fully focus on the moves that you are about to do.

As for the "how's" of warming up, there are two good ways, says Layne. You can choose the

She's Getting Nowhere Fast

When Barbara first saw those bins full of brightly colored, vinyl-clad dumbbells in a local sporting goods store, she just couldn't resist. She'd been wanting to do resistance training for a long time. On the sales clerk's advice, she bought 1-pound, 3-pound, and 5-pound sets, and she started lifting the moment she got home. Every day, after 30 minutes of aerobics, she did a great dumbbell routine that exercised every single part of her body. For the first few days, Barbara felt exhilarated. But now, 6 weeks later, she doesn't seem to be making any progress. Her muscles don't seem firmer, and she doesn't feel much stronger, even though she's doing endless repetitions of each exercise. Why isn't all of this weight lifting helping her?

Give Barbara credit for enthusiasm. Unfortunately, enthusiasm alone won't tone her muscles or make them stronger. Challenging them will. Barbara's light-weight, high-rep, everyday workouts clearly aren't doing that.

Lifting weights isn't supposed to hurt, but it's not supposed to be effortless, either. Barbara was right to start off at low weights, but in order to properly work a muscle, the weight should be heavy enough to make 8 to 12 repetitions, in good form, a challenge.

This brings us to another thing that's holding Barbara back. Barbara may have heard that using light weights with lots of repetitions is a way to avoid bulk as you tone. But her concern is misguided. Women simply won't bulk up the way some men do, because our hormones have other plans.

Barbara's daily full-body weight session is also sabotaging her efforts. If you keep training the same muscle group on consecutive days, you won't see results. That's because you're breaking down muscle tissue without giving it the 48 hours of recovery time that it needs to repair itself and adapt by getting stronger. She should work only her upper body one day and only her lower body the next.

Expert Consulted
Renee Cloe
Certified personal trainer
Cofounder of the Fitness Jumpsite Web site

one that works for you, depending on how much time you have to spare.

The first warmup method is simple, and it generates heat throughout your body: Just get moving for 5 minutes. You can do this by walking (either on a treadmill, around the block, or even in place) or climbing some stairs. The idea is not to burn calories or break a sweat—you're warming up on the inside more than anywhere else.

The second technique that Layne recommends is more specific. Instead of warming up your entire body at once, you can warm up bit by bit as you do your workout. Just go through the motions—the weight-lifting exercises—that you plan to do, but use only half of your normal amount of weight. For example, if your first exercises are biceps curls with a 5-pound weight, you would start with one warmup set of curls using only a 2- or 3-pound weight. After the warmup set, do your "real" set (or sets) of curls. Then move on to the warmup set for your next exercise.

Whether you decide to warm up with walking or another light activity, or by doing a run-through set of each exercise, what matters most is that you do it religiously, says Layne. Warming up properly is the first step of an injury-free, results-oriented workout.

The Form's the Thing

You've probably heard about exercising "to failure"—lifting until you reach the point where your muscles can no longer move a certain weight even one more time. A better way to lift, says Layne, is to focus on form. This means aiming to do each repetition of an exercise perfectly. When you start getting sloppy and find it hard to maintain good form, it's time to move on to the next exercise. Signs of good form include:

- Exhaling through your mouth on exertion (when you're actually lifting the weight rather than letting it back down)
- Moving your muscle through its entire range of motion (by moving the weights all the way up and all the way down for every exercise)
- Keeping your spine and neck in alignment and your body symmetrical (using good posture; keeping your shoulders relaxed and in-line and your spine straight)
- Being able to maintain a stable torso (when your body begins to tremble and quiver, you can bet that form is going away)

When you concentrate on form, you can't predict how many reps you will do. So while the directions for each exercise recommend a number to aim for, you should start with an open mind. "One good repetition with solid form is worth more than 10 fast and sloppy ones," says Karen Andes, author of several books on mind-body fitness and a certified personal trainer at Nautilus of Marin in San Rafael, California.

Like good music, good form requires rhythm. For optimal training effect and the best results possible, Layne recommends a

BALLET: BUILDING A MORE INTELLIGENT BODY

Rhythmic piano music fills the air as graceful arms lift and lower and elegant legs circle and extend. In a ballet performance, physical grace is the artistic expression of underlying muscular strength. Without toned thigh, shoulder, and abdominal muscles, ballet movements that seem to defy gravity simply would not be possible.

If you're already a dancer, you'll be glad to know that resistance training can give your performance an edge. "It definitely fills in the areas that dance doesn't reach," says Karen Andes, author of several books on mind-body fitness and a certified personal trainer at Nautilus of Marin in San Rafael, California. For example, hamstring curls build greater strength in the backs of your thighs than ballet alone, she says.

For the larger percentage of women who weight train but don't dance, ballet moves can fit right in. They make an ideal cross-training choice that provides toning benefits, according to Andes. In ballet, resistance is provided in the form of your own body weight rather than in dumbbells or weight plates. When a ballerina does a plié, which is really a type of squat, her torso weight supplies the resistance that her inner thighs have to work against as they bend and straighten.

Ballet brings other benefits to your weight training as well. "Adding ballet to a toning program teaches proper placement, better alignment, and heightened body awareness," says Andes. "Dance is good training for making your body more intelligent overall." This new intelligence makes injury less likely and graceful aging a sure thing.

specific lifting rhythm: Lift, or exert force, to a count of two; come to a complete stop for one count; then lower or return to where you started for a slow count of four. This method minimizes momentum (so there's less chance of "cheating") and will make your muscles more fit than quicker lifting and lowering will. For some moves where the range of motion is much smaller, such as abdominal exercises or leg/arm extensions, the recommended pattern is shorter: Lift for two; hold for one; lower for two.

The dance exercises presented in each chapter also require attention to form. But since you won't be using dumbbells, proper form is somewhat different. Here are Andes's tips for getting the most out of each ballet-type move.

Stand tall. For all standing dance exercises, you want to feel as if you are being gently pulled up toward the ceiling from a point at the very top of your head. "Before you even go down, you lift up a bit."

Sink down. At the same time that your body is pulling upward, you also need to use your leg muscles to push your feet into the floor. For example, a plié has both lifting and pushing forces working at the same time. "Properly done, there should be internal dynamic resistance going on in your body."

Keep your hands elegant. Allow your hands to gently curve toward the floor in a relaxed and graceful way. This will eliminate unnecessary muscle tension in your arms as well as in your hands and wrists.

Extend your neck. Do your best to keep your neck free of tension. "Your shoulders should be down at all times so you have the longest neck possible."

Do the Numbers: Reps, Sets, and When to Take a Break

Resistance training centers around repetitions of single movements that are known in weight-

---

FORGET ABOUT IT: MOVES THAT DO MORE HARM THAN GOOD

In the realm of resistance training, some exercises are notoriously shunned by personal trainers but are still believed to be effective by many women who work out.

"I'm surprised we even have to mention some of the more classic ones, but we do," says Karen Andes, author of several books on mind-body fitness and a certified personal trainer at Nautilus of Marin in San Rafael, California. In some cases, the moves are actually dangerous—potentially harmful to your muscles or joints. Others are simply a waste of time and won't actually boost your strength, regardless of how diligently you do them. Read on for the scoop on the "Forget about It Four."

1. Hurdler's stretch. In this stretch, one leg is extended out in front of you, and the other is bent at the knee with your inner thigh on the floor and your heel behind your body. You may do this to stretch the quadriceps and hip flexor on your bent leg and to target the hamstrings on your extended leg. However, this posture dangerously stretches the ligaments in the front of the knee that is bent, twists your kneecap out of alignment, and crushes the meniscus in the back of your knee. Just about any other stretch for those muscle groups is a safer alternative, says Andes.

2. Classic situps. Doing classic situps that bring you to a full sitting position transfers the work to your back and hip-flexor muscles, making this move basically useless

---

lifting circles as reps. The definition of a repetition is basically one complete movement through the entire range of motion for the muscle being worked.

Remember, the number of repetitions suggested under the goal-specific directions for each exercise is something to ultimately shoot for, but always use the above guidelines on proper form to guarantee that you're making every rep count. Maintaining proper form may mean doing fewer

as well as dangerous for your lower back. Also, yanking your body upright uses momentum, not muscle, and again compromises your lower back. Focused crunches where you raise only your head and shoulders off the floor are safer than full situps. And Pilates-style "roll-ups" and "roll-downs," which peel your spine off and onto the floor in a super slow-motion situp, are an excellent advanced option.

3. Step-forward lunge. "This is the move I hate most in the world, and many people still do it," says Andes. Lunging while stepping forward with one leg combines a forward force with a downward pressure. Both dangerous impulses end up in your kneecap. To protect your knees, do a lunge in place or a backward-stepping lunge, instead. Safer lunges are done with a stable torso, your knees over your ankles (not over your toes), and your front heel on the floor.

4. Overhead military press or pull-down done behind your head. This one is a definite "shouldn't" for your shoulders. Pressing a barbell or weight-machine handle from a behind-the-head position puts your shoulder rotator-cuff muscles as well as various tendons and ligaments at great risk of injury. It can also be dangerous to pull the bar behind your head, as in a lat pull-down. It's much safer and just as effective to pull the bar down in front of your chest. For shoulder presses with dumbbells or machine handles, place the weights or handles directly over your shoulders. When using a bar, press the bar from your chest over your head.

cording to the American College of Sports Medicine. But the number of sets that you will actually be doing when you use this book depends on your individual starting strength as well as on the goal that you've chosen.

Although it may not seem to make sense, for muscle to build maximum strength, rest days are absolutely necessary. That's because resistance training actually causes microscopic damage to muscle tissue. The healing that happens at the cellular level is what prompts muscle to grow and get stronger—the tissues are actually preparing for the next challenging workout that they'll have to face.

Muscle heals itself very quickly, says Layne. "A good 48 hours is really all it takes." So, in the basic toning program offered in this book, you will not be doing any back-to-back lifting for the same muscle group. There will always be at least one rest day, and sometimes two, in between workouts. On those days off, it's a good idea to stay active with aerobic exercise to both speed muscle healing and help you continue to burn calories.

Keeping Track of It All

reps to start with—and that's just fine. "Your form will automatically improve as you begin to develop strength," says Layne. And as your form improves, the number of reps that you can do properly will go up. For now, let perfection be your guide.

A set is a group of repetitions. One set equals the number of reps that you can do in perfect succession. One set per exercise is the bare minimum to help you achieve muscular fitness, ac-

Some gyms supply cards that you can use to keep track of the exercises you do there. Often, books on weight training offer preprinted workout logs for you to copy and fill out as a way to keep track of your progress. But cookie-cutter forms don't really reflect the individual experience of each woman who begins a workout program, says Andes. Instead, she recommends that you make your own log using a plain old notebook that you dedicate to that purpose.

"Doing it yourself helps you learn more; you'll pick up the names of the exercises as well as the muscles you're working," she says. "And if you know what you are doing, you're going to do it better."

Keeping a workout diary is simple. Use one page or more per workout session. Along the left margin, list the names of the exercises and, in parentheses, the muscles that they work. Then, using a line for each move, record the number of reps that you do in good form and the amount of weight that you lift that day. "Because you remember more when you are first learning, the more information you record at the start, the better," says Andes. "After a while, the little details will become automatic, and you can just record the name of the exercise."

It makes good sense to devote a section of your journal to diet as well. Try tracking what you ate before your workout. You can use the information to determine if some foods make you feel better or worse as you train.

Finally, it's a good idea to jot down some brief notes pertaining to your mood and energy level each time you work out, says Andes. Over time, this will give you a clear picture of your overall progress—not only will your journal show your strength gains but you'll be able to reflect on improvements and fluctuations in emotional evenness and vitality as well.

Here's a quick list of items to include in your workout diary. (But remember, you can always customize your diary to include more.)

- ❧ Name of each exercise and muscles worked (use this book for that information)
- ❧ Pounds lifted
- ❧ Number of sets and reps
- ❧ Meals eaten before and after your workout
- ❧ Point in your menstrual cycle (counting the first day of your period as day one)
- ❧ General mood
- ❧ Energy level (you can use a scale of 1 to 10)

The Why's and How's of Stretching for Success

If warming up is the introduction to the book of toning, stretching is certainly the all-important final chapter. Even if you already consider yourself flexible—and women do tend to be more limber, in general, than men—stretching adds a lot to a toning regimen. "Regular stretching helps you avoid injury and allows you to maintain the full range of motion in all of your joints and muscles," says Layne. "It's a component of fitness in and of itself."

The stretches included in each chapter should be done together at the end of your workout, whether you've been toning or treadmilling, says Layne. The postexercise period is the time when your muscles are at their warmest and loosest.

You can start with the areas that are notoriously inflexible and that are contributors to lower-back pain—namely, your hamstrings and the muscles in your lower back, says Layne. Make sure that you target each major muscle group with at least one stretch during each stretching session.

The timing of a stretch is crucial to its effectiveness, says Layne. Your ultimate goal is to comfortably hold each stretch for a full 30 seconds. But that doesn't mean you should push yourself past your limits and grimace the whole way through. It's better to stretch for shorter time in a pain-free way.

"Initially, you should be able to hold a stretch for at least 20 seconds," says Layne. "If you can't, then you're probably overreaching or trying to push yourself too far. Ease back an inch or a few inches, until you find a comfortable place to hold the stretch." Remember, the idea is to relax and lengthen each muscle, not to tighten up or increase tension.

Diamonds Can Be *Your* Best Friend

Strength training can do more than improve your health and appearance. It can also make you better at other physical activities you enjoy. Whether your preference is bowling with the league at your local lanes or dancing to the swing of an orchestra on a Saturday night, you can find specific strength-training exercises that will give your performance a boost. Just look for the gems that fit your preference among the exercises in the chapters that follow. Here's the key:

BOW **BOWLING:** Front Squat (page 66), Seated Fly (page 102), Upright Row (page 106), External Shoulder Rotation (page 108), Triceps Kickback (page 116), Dumbbell Row (page 126)

CYC **CYCLING:** Leg Extension (page 46), Standing Leg Curl (page 48), Butt Sculptor (page 64), Step-Up (page 68), External Shoulder Rotation (page 108), Land Swim (page 124)

DAN **DANCING:** Butt Sculptor (page 64), Abdominal Crunch with Rotation (page 80), Pelvic Tilt (page 82), Reverse Curl (page 84), Modified Pushup (page 96), Land Swim (page 124)

GLF **GOLF:** Outer-Leg Lift (page 42), Front Squat (page 66), Abdominal Crunch with Rotation (page 80), Chest Fly (page 94), Upright Row (page 106), External Shoulder Rotation (page 108), Land Swim (page 124), Dumbbell Row (page 126)

SKI **SKIING:** Outer-Leg Lift (page 42), Inner-Leg Lift (page 44), Butt Sculptor (page 64), Abdominal Crunch with Rotation (page 80), Pelvic Tilt (page 82)

SB **SOFTBALL:** Outer-Leg Lift (page 42), Front Squat (page 66), Chest Fly (page 94), Seated Fly (page 102), Triceps Kickback (page 116), Pullover (page 128)

SWI **SWIMMING:** Seated Fly (page 102), Overhead Triceps Extension (page 118), Land Swim (page 124), Pullover (page 128)

TEN **TENNIS:** Abdominal Crunch with Rotation (page 80), Chest Fly (page 94), Modified Pushup (page 96), Upright Row (page 106), External Shoulder Rotation (page 108), Overhead Triceps Extension (page 118), Dumbbell Row (page 126), Pullover (page 128)

VOL **VOLLEYBALL:** Front Squat (page 66), Step-Up (page 68), Abdominal Crunch with Rotation (page 80), Reverse Curl (page 84), Modified Pushup (page 96), Seated Fly (page 102)

Making Your Toning Routine Less Than Routine

Here are four different programs you can apply to the exercises in the following chapters. Or you can mix and match the exercises to create your own routines and add life to your lifting.

BASIC I

Choose this efficient whole-body routine for the first 6 to 8 weeks of toning. Do it two or three times a week, on nonconsecutive days. To make the most of this routine, do the exercises in the order listed. This alternates between your upper and lower body, and moves from larger to smaller muscle groups.

1. Front Squat	page 66
2. Chest Press	page 92
3. Leg Extension	page 46
4. Upright Row	page 106
5. Standing Leg Curl	page 48
6. Seated Overhead Press	page 104
7. Calf Raise	page 56
8. External Shoulder Rotation	page 108
9. Pelvic Tilt	page 82
10. Land Swim	page 124

BASIC II

Use this slightly more advanced routine as an alternative to Basic I, after you've learned good technique and developed some muscle strength. Do it two to three times a week, on nonconsecutive days.

1. Step-Up	page 68
2. Chest Fly	page 94
3. Outer-Leg Lift	page 42
4. Inner-Leg Lift	page 44
5. Seated Fly	page 102
6. Toe Raise	page 58
7. Dumbbell Row	page 126
8. Overhead Triceps Extension	page 118
9. Arm Curl	page 114
10. Abdominal Crunch	page 78

PUSH-PULL

This program is more intense than Basic I or II. It is designed to work opposing muscle groups. This makes your muscles work harder—and become more fatigued, so they'll need more rest. Do it two or three times a week, on nonconsecutive days.

1. Leg Extension	page 46
2. Standing Leg Curl	page 48
3. Chest Press	page 92
4. Dumbbell Row	page 126
5. Outer-Leg Lift	page 42
6. Inner-Leg Lift	page 44
7. Pullover	page 128
8. Seated Fly	page 102
9. Abdominal Crunch with Rotation	page 80
10. Reverse Curl	page 84

SIMPLE SPLIT

This program is based on a three-day rotation: The first day targets your upper body and abdomen; the second day works your lower body and back; and the third day allows for rest. Begin the split again with the first-day routine. Build up a good base of strength and technique before you attempt this challenging program.

UPPER BODY AND ABDOMEN

1. Chest Press	page 92
2. Pullover	page 128
3. Chest Fly	page 94
4. Seated Overhead Press	page 104
5. Upright Row	page 106
6. Triceps Kickback	page 116
7. Arm Curl	page 114
8. External Shoulder Rotation	page 108
9. Reverse Curl	page 84
10. Abdominal Crunch with Rotation	page 80

LOWER BODY AND BACK

1. Front Squat	page 66
2. Step-Up	page 68
3. Butt Sculptor	page 64
4. Outer-Leg Lift	page 42
5. Inner-Leg Lift	page 44
6. Toe Raise	page 58
7. Calf Raise	page 56
8. Land Swim	page 124

The Thighs You Want

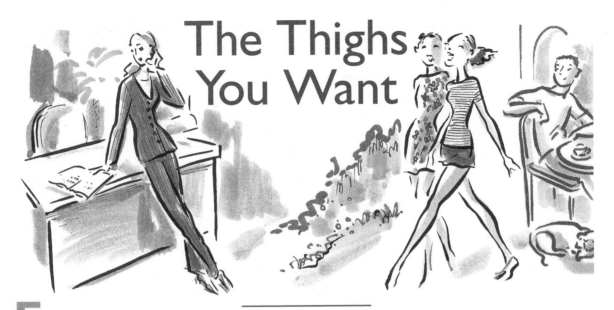

Everyone who wears miniskirts, raise your hand!

What, you haven't worn any kind of short skirt since Jimmy Carter was in office? You're not alone. The truth is, lots of women over 35 wouldn't dare wear skirts that are hemmed above the knee, for fear of revealing their thighs. In fact, when it comes to areas of the body that women want to slim down and shape up the most, the thighs have it.

Why are thighs so high on our "to-tone" lists? Because they're one area where women tend to store fat. Sure, a low-fat diet and aerobic exercise can help, but to firm up your thighs and give them a great shape, you have to do toning exercises as well.

Even when women *do* work out regularly, they often don't do the right exercises or lift heavy-enough weights to give their thighs more definition, says Jennifer Layne, an exercise physiologist at Tufts University in Boston. "Some women fear that their legs are going to get bigger if they target those muscles," she says. "That just isn't true."

The muscles in your thighs may take longer to tone than those in your upper body, but your ex-ercise perseverance is sure to pay off. "Having a stronger lower body is going to make everything in your life easier," Layne says. Lifting a heavy basket full of laundry off the floor. Running up the stairs after your 6-year-old. Fitting into those pants that are a bit snug.

Firmer thighs also mean healthier knees. When the muscles that attach to your knees are stronger, they're able to absorb the impact from your daily activities, so your knees undergo less wear and tear, Layne explains. Even women with moderate forms of arthritis of the knee, such as osteo-arthritis, have reduced pain and improved func-tion with strength-training exercises, she adds.

Before you start strapping on ankle weights, here's a quick anatomy lesson. Your thighs are made up of four major muscle groups. The largest are the quadriceps in the fronts of your thighs and the hamstrings in the backs of your thighs. Then there's the abductor muscles that stretch from your knees to your hips, along the outsides of your thighs. They help you move your legs out to the sides. Along your inner thighs run the adductor muscles, which help bring your legs together.

THE EXERCISES

Outer-Leg Lift

▶ WHAT IT DOES
Tones your outer thigh

▶ IT'S GOOD FOR:

  GLF golf

SKI skiing

SB softball

▶ GO FOR YOUR GOAL

Drop a Dress Size: *Two sets of 10 reps on each side, with up to 2-pound ankle weights*

Shape Up: *Three sets of 8 reps on each side, with 2- to 6-pound ankle weights*

Maintain: *Two to three sets of 8 to 12 reps on each side, with 6- to 10-pound ankle weights*

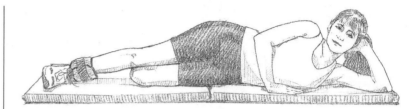

STEP 1: Strap an ankle weight on each ankle. Lie on a mat on your left side with your legs straight and together, one right on top of the other. Bend the lower part of your left leg back behind you, making sure to keep your hips and knees aligned. Support your head with your left arm, and place your right hand on the floor in front of you for balance.

Key things to remember
- Keep body in straight line
- Keep leg straight
- Point toes forward
- Balance with hand on floor
- Bend back lower leg
- Support head and neck

LISTEN TO YOUR BODY

To do the outer-leg lift correctly, you should move your leg from the hip and keep the rest of your body still, says exercise physiologist Jennifer Layne. Some people "cheat" by using their whole bodies to lift their legs. "They move their torsos, trunks, or stomachs instead of just their legs. Others lean so their bodies are no longer in straight lines, or they

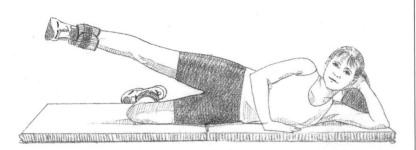

STEP 2: In a slow, controlled movement, take two counts to lift your top leg as high as you can without rotating your hip or making any abrupt secondary movements in an attempt to lift your leg higher. Keep your leg straight and your foot flat, with your toes pointed straight ahead. Hold your leg at the top of the move for one count, and then take four counts to lower it back to the starting position. Exhale as you raise your leg, and inhale as you lower it.

Repeat until you've competed one set, and then roll onto your right side and do a set with your other leg. Continue alternating legs between sets until you've completed all of the sets for your goal.

Key things to remember
- Keep foot flat, with toes pointed forward
- Don't lock knee
- Don't lean body forward or backward

▶ **TAKE IT TO THE MAX**
To give your outer thighs the maximum workout, gently push the heel of your top leg away from you before each repetition of the outer-leg lift. "That helps to straighten your leg and keep your foot in the correct position," says exercise physiologist Jennifer Layne. "It also makes the move slightly more intense."

roll back onto their buttocks," she says. Focus on keeping your body still and straight, and use only the muscles in your leg to lift it up.

If you find yourself rolling backward or forward, you may be trying to lift your leg too high, or you may need to decrease the amount of weight you're lifting while you master the technique, Layne says.

THE EXERCISES

Inner-Leg Lift

▶ **WHAT IT DOES**
Works your inner thigh

▶ **IT'S GOOD FOR:**

 skiing

▶ **GO FOR YOUR GOAL**

Drop a Dress Size: *Two sets of 10 reps on each side, with up to 2-pound ankle weights*

Shape Up: *Three sets of 8 reps on each side, with 2- to 6-pound ankle weights*

Maintain: *Two to three sets of 8 to 12 reps on each side, with 6- to 12-pound ankle weights*

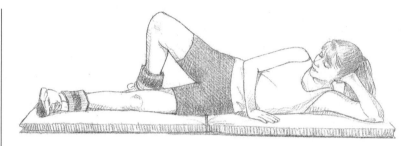

STEP 1: Fasten an ankle weight around each ankle. Lie on a mat on your left side with your left leg outstretched and your toes pointing forward. Bend your right knee and plant your right foot flat on the floor behind and parallel to your left leg. Your body should be in a straight line. You can prop your head up with your left arm or outstretch your arm and lay your head down on it. Place your right hand on the floor in front of you for balance.

Key things to remember
• Keep body in a straight line
• Balance with arm and back leg
• Keep leg straight
• Point toes forward

LISTEN TO YOUR BODY

One of the keys to doing the inner-leg lift correctly is to make sure that you're moving your leg from the hip and that that is *all* you're moving. If you find yourself rolling forward or backward onto your buttocks, or if you don't keep your torso still, that means you're using muscles other than those in your thigh to help lift your leg, says exercise physiologist Jennifer Layne.

Another common mistake that may cause a real pain in the neck later on is tensing up your neck muscles as you lift your leg. "This

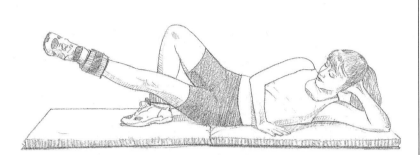

STEP 2: Exhale as you take two counts to lift your left leg off the floor, keeping your leg straight and your foot flat. Raise your leg as high as you comfortably can without rocking your body forward or backward. Hold your leg at the top of the lift for one count, and then inhale for four counts as you lower your leg back to the starting position.

Repeat until you've completed one set, then roll over onto your right side and do a set with your right leg. Continue alternating legs between sets until you've completed all of the sets for your goal.

Key things to remember
- Keep foot flat
- Keep upper body still
- Keep leg straight

tends to happen when people lift heavier weights," Layne says. So concentrate on keeping your neck relaxed as you do the move.

If you're having a tough time keeping your balance, make this minor adjustment: Roll back about an inch onto your buttock. "That will help keep you steady and give you more room to lift your leg," Layne says. Just make sure that you stay in that position as you do the move, she adds. Don't roll back as you lift and then roll forward as you lower. "This position is okay for beginners, but your goal is to do the move while lying on your side with your top hip as far forward as possible," Layne says.

▶ **TAKE IT
TO THE MAX**
You can make the inner-leg lift a more advanced exercise by changing your position. Lie on your back with your legs straight up in the air so that from a side view your torso and trunk form an L. Place your hands, palms down, under your buttocks to help keep your lower back pressed firmly against the floor. Keep your feet flat so your toes point toward your torso. Then open your legs so they make a V. Hold for one count and slowly bring your legs back together. Your legs should remain straight during the move, with your knees just short of being locked. Start out by opening your legs about 12 inches, and work up to 18 to 24 inches. To get the maximum workout, do the move with the appropriate ankle weights for your goal.

Leg Extension

▶ **WHAT IT DOES**
Targets your quadriceps

▶ **IT'S GOOD FOR:**

 cycling

▶ **GO FOR YOUR GOAL**

Drop a Dress Size: *Two sets of 10 reps each with 3- to 5-pound ankle weights*

Shape Up: *Three sets of 8 reps each with 5- to 10-pound ankle weights*

Maintain: *Two to three sets of 8 to 12 reps each with 10- to 20-pound ankle weights*

STEP 1: Strap an ankle weight onto each ankle. Sit all the way back on a table or chair with your knees bent so that your thighs and lower legs form a 90-degree angle. The edge of the table should go right up to your knees so your thighs are entirely supported. Place your feet about shoulder-width apart and make sure the table is high enough so that your toes barely touch the floor. If necessary, you can boost yourself up by placing a phone book on the table. Or try doing the exercise seated on your washer or dryer. Use a step stool or chair to get onto the machine. Then strap on your ankle weights and sit with the bend of your knee at the edge of the washer or dryer so that your thighs are fully supported. Place your hands on your thighs.

Key things to remember
• Sit against chair back
• Keep knees at edge of chair
• Touch floor with toes
• Bend knees at 90-degree angle

LISTEN TO YOUR BODY

If you feel pain or discomfort in your knee when doing a leg extension, one of three things may be the cause. First, you may be locking your knee so you can lift your leg higher. "Don't worry if your leg isn't completely straight or as high as shown in the picture," says exercise physiologist Jennifer Layne. "Work at your own level of ability and your own range of motion."

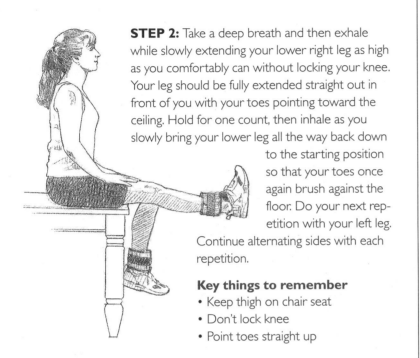

STEP 2: Take a deep breath and then exhale while slowly extending your lower right leg as high as you comfortably can without locking your knee. Your leg should be fully extended straight out in front of you with your toes pointing toward the ceiling. Hold for one count, then inhale as you slowly bring your lower leg all the way back down to the starting position so that your toes once again brush against the floor. Do your next repetition with your left leg. Continue alternating sides with each repetition.

Key things to remember
• Keep thigh on chair seat
• Don't lock knee
• Point toes straight up

▶ **TAKE IT TO THE MAX**
Once you've mastered the leg extension, the only safe way to make it more difficult is to use heavier weights. Do *not* lift both legs at the same time when using ankle weights, cautions exercise physiologist Jennifer Layne. Machines at the gym are designed so that you can safely lift both legs, but when you're wearing ankle weights, there is too much pressure on your lumbar spine and you may suffer an injury, she says.

A second possibility is that you're lifting your thigh slightly off the chair as you raise your leg to the extended position. "Lifting your thigh can compress your knee joint," Layne says, "and that's something you certainly do not want to do."

Third, your knees may be bothering you if the seat of the chair does not extend all the way to your knees. When your thighs are not entirely supported by the seat, you put stress on your knees, Layne says.

THE EXERCISES

Standing Leg Curl

▶ **WHAT IT DOES**
Strengthens your hamstrings

▶ **IT'S GOOD FOR:**

 cycling

▶ **GO FOR YOUR GOAL**
Drop a Dress Size: *Two sets of 10 reps on each side, without weights, for one or two sessions; then two sets of 10 reps on each side, with 2- to 4-pound ankle weights*

Shape Up: *Three sets of 8 reps on each side, with 4- to 6-pound ankle weights*

Maintain: *Two to three sets of 8 to 12 reps on each side, with 6- to 10-pound ankle weights*

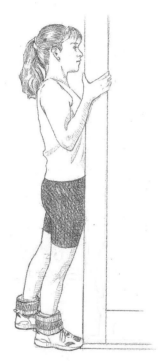

STEP 1: If you're using weights for this exercise, strap an ankle weight onto each ankle. Stand with good posture with the fronts of your right hip and thigh stabilized against a doorjamb or your refrigerator. Plant your feet flat on the floor a few inches apart, with your left foot a few inches behind your right foot. Hold on to the doorjamb or refrigerator handle for support.

Key things to remember
- Keep body in straight line
- Stand with feet parallel, one behind the other
- Press fronts of hip and thigh against doorjamb

 LISTEN TO YOUR BODY

   If the muscles in your butt feel like they're getting a workout, that means you're using those muscles instead of your hamstrings to help you do the standing leg curl, says exercise physiologist Jennifer Layne. Standing against a doorjamb or refrigerator helps to isolate your hamstrings and prevents you from using other muscles to do the exercise, but you still need to concentrate on using just your hamstrings and moving only your lower leg. "Everything else—your thigh, butt, and the rest of your body—

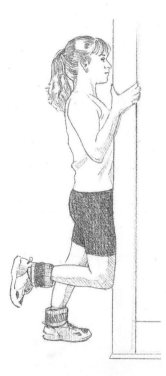

STEP 2: Keeping your right hip and thigh firmly against the doorjamb, bend your right knee and slowly lift your lower right leg up behind you so that it's parallel to the floor and your toes point down. Avoid bringing your knee forward or backward—it should remain pressed against the doorjamb. Hold this position for one count. Then take four counts to lower your leg back to the starting position. Remember to exhale as you lift and inhale as you lower.

After completing one set with your right leg, do a set with your left. Continue alternating legs until you finish all of your sets.

Key things to remember
• Keep thigh pressed against doorjamb
• Keep knee in line with hip
• Don't arch back
• Point toes down
• Bend knee at 90-degree angle

▶ **TAKE IT
TO THE MAX**
You can work your hamstrings even harder by not giving them a break between repetitions of the standing leg curl, says exercise physiologist Jennifer Layne. When you bring your lower leg back down to the floor after a rep, just touch your toes to the floor instead of putting your whole foot down and sliding it forward.

should remain perfectly still," Layne explains. It's okay if you feel some effort in the thigh of the leg that's supporting your weight, she adds.

To prevent lower-back strain, make sure you don't arch your back when you lift your leg behind you, Layne cautions.

If you get a cramp or charley horse in your leg, stop exercising and take a short break. The pain means the exercise is too intense. Lower the intensity by lightening each ankle weight by 1 to 2 pounds. Or do half a set on one leg, then switch and do half on the other. Then go back to the first leg and finish up your set, and so on.

THE EXERCISES

Degagé First-Position Plié to Second

▶ **WHAT IT DOES**
Strengthens your quadri-
ceps and inner thighs

▶ **GO FOR YOUR GOAL**
Drop a Dress Size: *Two
to four reps on each side*

Shape Up: *Four to six
reps on each side*

Maintain: *Six to eight
reps on each side*

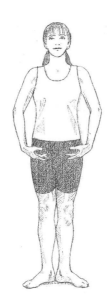

STEP 1: Start in ballet first position, with your
toes turned to 2 and 10 o'clock and with proper
posture, as shown. Your thighs, calves, and heels
should touch, and your abs and buttocks should
be tight. Press your shoulders down and place
your hands (with rounded arms) in front of your
thighs. You should move at a pace that is slow
enough to allow you to feel completely in control
of your muscles during the exercise. If necessary,
hold on to the back of a chair for balance.

Key things to remember
• Stand with heels together
• Tighten abs
• Squeeze buttocks
• Press shoulders down

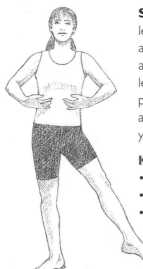

STEP 2: Transfer your weight to your right
leg as you lift your left leg forward off the floor
at about a 45-degree angle. Keep your torso
and supporting leg as straight as possible. Your
left leg should be straight, with your toes
pointed toward the floor. Raise your arms up
along the midline of your body to just below
your chest.

Key things to remember
• Keep body straight
• Point toes
• Round hands below chest

STEP 3: Reach out to the side with your left leg and plant your left foot on the floor so that your heels are sep-arated by 1 ½ to 2 times the width of your hips. Your feet should be pointed to 2 and 10 o'clock. This is ballet second position. Bend your knees and lower your body into a plié as deeply as you can while maintaining a vertical torso, keeping your knees directly over your ankles (not over your toes). Stretch your arms straight out to your sides at shoulder height. Then return to ballet first position by squeezing your legs together and dragging your right leg back to your left. Bring your arms down so they are rounded, with your hands in front of your thighs. Hold each position for a slow to moderate two counts, for a total of eight counts. Repeat until you have completed all of the reps for your goal, then do the appropriate number of reps with your right leg.

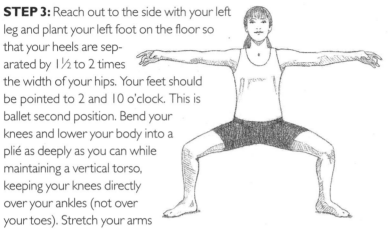

Key things to remember
• Don't lift heels
• Keep knees over ankles
• Keep feet about twice your hip-width apart
• Hold arms straight out

▶ **TAKE IT TO THE MAX**
You can work your quads and inner thighs even harder with the degagé first-position plié to second by using a wider stance for the plié. The farther apart your feet are, the deeper you can go into the plié. Just make sure your knees are di-rectly above your ankles when you're at the bottom of the move, cau-tions certified personal trainer Karen Andes.

LISTEN TO YOUR BODY

If your knees feel as though they're doing most of the work during the degagé first-position plié to second, double-check your form. When you start out in ballet first position and when you bend into the plié, make sure your toes point to 2 and 10 o'clock. "People tend to overdo it and turn their feet to 3 and 9 o'clock, which is hard on the knees," says certified personal trainer Karen Andes. When you lower into the plié, make sure your knees stay in line with your ankles.

If you feel pain, weakness, or discomfort in the hip of your supporting leg when the other leg is lifted, that means you're leaning into your hip too much. To fix your form, keep your supporting leg and torso as straight as possible.

THE STRETCHES

Quadriceps Stretch

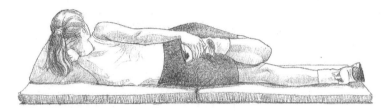

▶ **WHAT IT DOES**
Lengthens the muscles in the fronts of the thighs

▶ **HOW TO DO IT**
Lie on your left side with your legs straight and together, one right on top of the other. Then bend the knee of your top leg so your foot comes back toward your buttocks. Grasp your foot and pull your heel toward your butt. At the same time, push your buttocks and hip forward to resist the backward movement of your foot and to increase the stretch. Just make sure to keep your hips and knees in line with each other. You should feel a comfortable stretch in the front of your thigh. Hold the stretch for 30 seconds, and then stretch the other leg.

Key things to remember
- Keep body straight
- Align thighs and knees
- Pull foot in, not up
- Push hip forward; don't let it move back

ME? EXERCISING TOO MUCH?

For most women, the opposite is true: We exercise too little. But women who become fanatical about it, who can't take a day off, or who start training for a race or some other event can set themselves up for overtraining syndrome.

"You're tired all the time and you begin to hate exercising," says Jean Reeve, Ph.D., a triathlete and an associate professor of physical education at Southern Utah University in Cedar City. Overtraining can be insidious because your decline in performance may make you push yourself even harder, when what your body really needs is rest.

Other symptoms of overdoing it: aches and pains you just can't shake off; irritability; persistent flu-like symptoms, including a mild headache or a runny nose; a marked decrease in appetite; a troubled sleep pattern; or an elevated heart rate, even at rest.

If you fit this bill, start with 1 or 2 full weeks off from exercise, then go from there, Dr. Reeve says. Once you start feeling up to it, slowly increase the intensity of your routine again, she says. "And remember, you don't have to stay in peak shape all the time. Not even the pros do that."

THE STRETCHES

Seated Hamstring Stretch

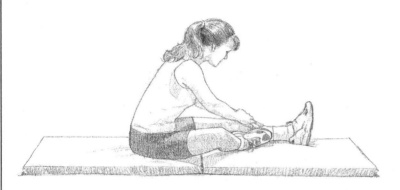

▶ WHAT IT DOES

Stretches the muscles in the back of your thigh

▶ HOW TO DO IT

Sit on the floor with your left leg extended straight out in front of you and your right leg bent so that the sole of your right foot rests against your left calf. Bend forward from your left hip only as far you can without rounding your back. You should feel the stretch in the back of your left thigh and in the back of your left lower leg. Hold for 30 seconds. Sit up slowly, and then stretch your other hamstring.

Key things to remember

- Point toes up
- Keep back straight
- Bend from hips, not waist
- Keep leg straight
- Keep chest lifted

▶ DESKTOP TRAINER

Seated Leg Lift

Here's a way to give your thighs a quick workout at work. Sit all the way back in your chair with your feet flat on the floor. Your arms can be down at your sides or on the armrests of the chair. Raise your right lower leg so that your right leg is straight and fully extended, just short of locking your knee, with your toes pointing upward. Keeping it straight, raise your entire right leg, from your thigh to your toes, as high as you can off the chair. Be careful to not lock your knee as you lift your leg. Hold for one count. Lower your leg back to the starting position and repeat. Do 8 to 12 reps with your right leg, and then switch and do 8 to 12 reps with your left.

REAL-LIFE SCENARIO

Her Thighs Are Growing, Rather Than Slimming

Before Lucille opened the box that was lying on her living room floor, she let her fingers trace its shape gingerly, as if it were something strange and wonderful. It had taken her a long time to build up the courage to buy this thing. She hadn't exercised in years, and she was 46 now. Maybe it was too late to start. But she had seen this thing so many times in the department store, heard so much about it, and even imagined herself on it. So she had finally broken down, pulled out her credit card, and made one her very own. An aerobic step. This was to be the answer to all of that weight that she had put on her lower body over the past decade. In no time, she was going up and down like a born climber and dreaming about the toned hips, butt, and thighs that she was going to have. Gradually, her legs grew stronger. She raised the height of the step, then raised it again. To supplement her workout, she took her bicycle out of the garage and began taking to the hills on the weekends. Now she feels better than ever, except for one problem: Her thighs haven't gotten smaller. They've gotten bigger. What can she do?

Lucille has found out the hard way that stronger doesn't necessarily mean slimmer. To make her thighs smaller, she needs to build muscle *and* burn fat. Lucille may be missing out on the fat-burning benefits of aerobic exercise by making her workouts too challenging. Because she has raised her step twice, it's probably quite high off the ground. Yet she's still a beginner when it comes to exercise, so it's likely that she can't maintain a high intensity for very long when doing her step routine.

As for her weekend bike ride, cycling through hilly terrain isn't the best way to lose weight, either. Sure, these tough workouts have made her legs stronger. Lucille has built muscle—but that muscle is probably hidden under a layer of fat.

The way for Lucille to shrink her thighs is to lower the aerobic step to a height where she can maintain a moderate intensity for 30 minutes. She can gauge her intensity by wearing layers such as a T-shirt and a sweatshirt at the start of her routine. Once she has broken a sweat and needs to take off her top layer, she will know that that is the intensity she needs to maintain for 30 minutes.

After she has worked out at that intensity for 20 minutes, her body's calorie-burning furnace will switch from burning mostly carbohydrates to mostly fat, so the last 10 minutes of her workout will be primarily fat-burning. This type of workout—lower intensity for a longer duration—builds endurance rather than strength and is much more effective at getting rid of unwanted fat.

Lucille may want to take her bike out on flatter surfaces as well. Some hills are fine, but going through rough terrain is more like aerobic interval training, which also is great for building muscle but not so great for losing weight. She should use the same 30-minutes-at-a-somewhat-hard-intensity guideline for her bike rides as well.

Expert Consulted
Iona Passik
Certified personal trainer and master trainer and presenter for Spinning, the original indoor
     cycling program
New York Sports Club
New York City

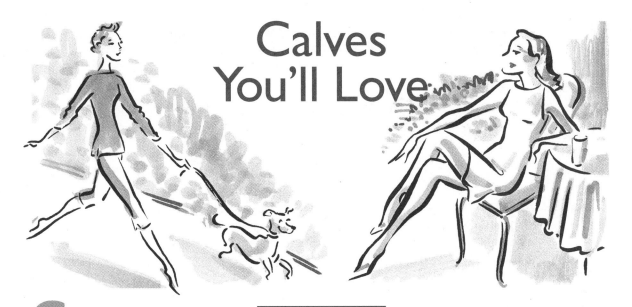

Calves You'll Love

Calves. You don't need to be a ballerina or an Olympic diver to appreciate what strong calves can do for you. You use them every time you stand up, take a step, climb a flight of stairs, or press on a brake pedal. Add up all that stepping and braking, and the average healthy woman contracts her calves more than 10,000 times a day.

And that's not all. Your calf muscles also help support your posture, says Jennifer Layne, an exercise physiologist at Tufts University in Boston.

Tone your calves, and you'll not only be able to do all that walking and stairclimbing with less effort but you'll also develop shapely lower legs that you'll be proud to pull panty hose over. Here's how.

You need to tone two muscles—the gastrocnemius, found at the fattest part of your calf, and the soleus, which lies underneath the gastrocnemius. Both muscles help you go up on your toes to reach that rarely used wooden salad bowl from the top shelf, point your toes, and push off your front foot when you walk or run.

To create muscle balance—which is important for preventing injuries—you also need to work the front of your lower legs, Layne says. The anterior tibial stretches from your knee to your ankle in the front of your leg and is the muscle you use when you flex your foot toward you. Strengthening this muscle helps prevent shinsplints—a strain of the long flexor muscle of the toes that causes pain to shoot down your shin bone—during other activities. Shinsplints can result from suddenly intensifying your activity, Layne says, so if you're running or walking as part of a daily workout, be careful not to increase your speed or distance too much from day to day. Also, be careful of taking on steep, uphill grades before you're ready.

The exercises below work the soleus, gastrocnemius, and tibialis anterior muscles to give you shapely legs that you won't want to hide under a long skirt. Having strong lower legs also improves your balance and agility and makes you less prone to falls, Layne says. Add the following exercises to your fitness routine now, and you'll have lovelier legs in 6 to 8 weeks.

THE EXERCISES

Calf Raise

▶ **WHAT IT DOES**
Gives your calf muscles
more definition

▶ **IT'S GOOD FOR:**
All sports

▶ **GO FOR YOUR GOAL**

Drop a Dress Size: *Two
sets of 10 reps on the floor
for 2 to 4 weeks; then two
sets of 10 reps on the stairs
without weights*

Shape Up: *Three sets of
8 reps on the stairs with
one 5- to 8-pound dumbbell*

Maintain: *Two to three
sets of 8 to 12 reps on the
stairs with one 8- to 15-
pound dumbbell*

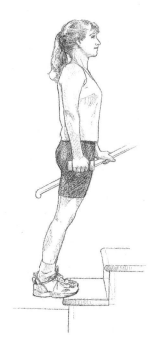

STEP 1: Beginners should try this exercise
on the floor first. Stand up straight with
your feet about hip-width apart, flat on the
floor. You can support yourself by touching
a wall lightly with your fingertips. Once
you've mastered this exercise on the floor,
you can move to the stairs.

   Stand on the bottom step of a staircase
and hold on to the railing with one hand for
support. If there is no staircase where you
do your workout, you can stand on an aerobic step bench and hold on to a countertop at your side. Start by placing the front
of both feet on the step so that the balls of
your feet are on the step's edge and your
toes point forward. The heels of your feet
should hang off the back, below the level of
the step. If you're using weights, hold the
dumbbell straight down at your side with
your free hand.

Key things to remember
• Don't lock knees
• Don't lean forward
• Put balls of feet at edge of step
• Keep feet parallel with each other

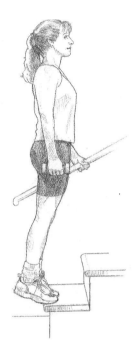

STEP 2: Without locking your knees or leaning forward, lift up onto your toes as high as you can. Hold for one count, then return to the starting position by slowly lowering your heels below the level of the step. Repeat.

Key things to remember

• Don't lock knees
• Don't lean forward
• Look straight ahead
• Go up on toes as far as you can

▶ **TAKE IT
TO THE MAX**
To take the calf-raise exercise to the next level, try working one calf at a time. Simply bend one leg at the knee so that leg is behind you. Then do the calf raise the same way as before—but this time you'll be using only one leg to support your weight. After completing your sets, switch legs. If you do the exercise with a dumbbell, you may need to use a lighter weight for this variation, says exercise physiologist Jennifer Layne.

LISTEN TO YOUR BODY

To get the most out of the calf raise, remember two key points: First, do the move slowly. Hold for one count when you're up on your toes, then gradually lower. The second point to watch out for is that you should not lock your knees in place and just raise up and down on your toes. "That's one of the most common mistakes I see when people do this exercise," says exercise physiologist Jennifer Layne. "Your legs should be straight, but your knees should not be locked. It's a good idea to do a mental check between reps to make sure you're not locking them."

If you're having trouble keeping your balance, move more of your feet onto the step or do the exercise on the floor, Layne suggests.

A cramp in your calves means you need to rest. Do only half of the reps, then walk around or do another exercise and come back and finish your set later, Layne says.

THE EXERCISES

Toe Raise

▶ **WHAT IT DOES**
Works the calves and the tibialis anterior muscles in the fronts of your lower legs

▶ **IT'S GOOD FOR:**
All sports

▶ **GO FOR YOUR GOAL**

Drop a Dress Size: *Two sets of 10 reps with up to 5-pound ankle weights*

Shape Up: *Three sets of 8 reps with 5- to 10-pound ankle weights*

Maintain: *Two to three sets of 8 to 12 reps with 10- to 20-pound ankle weights*

STEP 1: Sit in a chair with your feet flat on the floor. Strap ankle weights around your feet so they're on top of your shoelaces. Make sure your back is against the back of the chair. Hold on to the arms of the chair with your hands, or rest your arms on your thighs. To start, extend your legs slightly so that your heels are 3 to 4 inches off the floor, and point your toes away from you as far as you can. Hold for one count.

Key things to remember
- Sit against chair back
- Keep knees slightly bent
- Point toes
- Hold heels 3 to 4 inches off floor

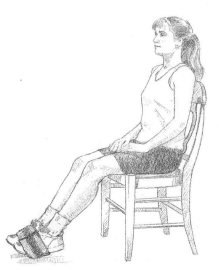

 LISTEN TO YOUR BODY

When you do the toe raise, you may feel like the tops of your thighs are getting a workout as well because you're using your quadriceps to keep your legs raised off the floor. If you need to give your quads a break, put your feet down on the floor and rest after 5 reps, or lower your legs so they're only about 2 inches off the floor while you do the move, suggests exercise physiologist Jennifer Layne.

If you feel the effort in your knees, check to make sure they aren't locked. No matter how many inches you lift your legs off the floor,

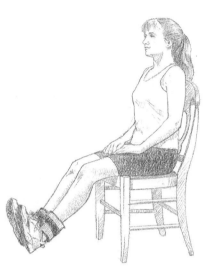

STEP 2: While keeping your feet raised off the floor, pull your toes toward you while pushing your heels away. Your legs should not move. Hold for one count. Return to the starting position by flexing your toes away from you. Repeat.

Key things to remember

• Flex toes
• Sit against chair back
• Keep knees slightly bent

▶ TAKE IT
TO THE MAX
The advanced exerciser can make the toe-raise move more challenging by lifting her legs higher off the floor so that they're almost fully extended.

your knees should be slightly bent, Layne says. Another thing that could cause discomfort in your knees is the wrong chair. The seat of the chair should be deep enough to support your entire thigh, she says. That means the edge of the seat should extend all the way to your knees. Not sitting completely back in the chair can also put strain on your knees as well as on your lower back, Layne adds.

If your feet wobble or rotate out to the sides as you flex them, try decreasing your weights by about 2 pounds, Layne says. The weights should feel challenging, but you should be able to control the movement of your feet, keeping them in a straight line.

Plié Relevé

▶ **WHAT IT DOES**
Strengthens your soleus and gastrocnemius muscles

▶ **GO FOR YOUR GOAL**
Drop a Dress Size: *6 to 12 reps*
Shape Up: *16 reps*
Maintain: *24 reps*

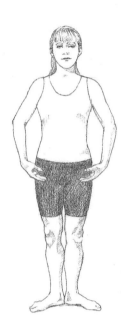

STEP 1: Start in ballet first position, with your toes turned to 2 and 10 o'clock and with proper posture, as shown. Your thighs, calves, and heels should touch, and your abs and buttocks should be tight. Press your shoulders down and hold your hands in front of your thighs, with your elbows slightly rounded. If necessary, hold on to the back of a chair for balance.

Key things to remember
• Stand with heels together
• Tighten abs
• Squeeze buttocks
• Press shoulders down

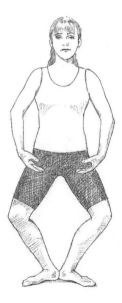

STEP 2: In a slow, fluid movement, bend your knees and lower your body into a demi-plié with your knees over your toes and your heels flat on the floor. Your knees should not extend beyond your toes. As you lower, create internal resistance by contracting your inner thighs as if you were squeezing a balloon between them. Keep your abs and buttocks tight. Return to the starting position by pressing down on your heels and pushing your thighs, knees, and calves back together.

Key things to remember
• Don't lift heels
• Maintain posture
• Contract inner thighs
• Keep knees over (not beyond) toes

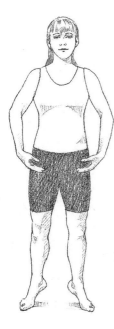

STEP 3: Squeeze your buttocks and press your inner thighs together as you slowly lift up your heels so that your weight is on the balls of your feet. This pose is known as relevé. Return once again to ballet first position by slowly coming back down out of the relevé. You should hold each pose for one or two counts. Repeat.

Key things to remember
- Squeeze buttocks
- Press inner thighs together
- Balance on balls of feet

▶ **TAKE IT TO THE MAX**

To make the plié relevé more challenging, pick up the pace. "Calves are stubborn muscles," says certified personal trainer Karen Andes. Because calves contain very densely woven, strong muscles, going faster usually means doing more total reps. And more reps equals more work for your calves. "Just make sure you don't sacrifice form for speed," says Andes.

LISTEN TO YOUR BODY

The trick to doing the plié relevé the right way is to ease down slowly from the relevé. "If you bounce down too hard, your whole body will be jarred as if you have bad shock absorbers in your knees, hips, and spine," says certified personal trainer Karen Andes.

If you're having trouble keeping your balance, make sure to squeeze your buttocks together and keep your eyes focused on something in front of you as you do the move. It may help to imagine your body sliding up and down an internal pole. Place your emphasis on the downward move rather than the upward lift, Andes says, so it's as if you go up just to come back down.

▶ THE STRETCHES

Calf Stretch

▶ **DESKTOP TRAINER**

Air Writer

Here's a discrete calf exercise that you can do at your desk. Sit in the same position as you would to do the toe-raise exercise on page 58. Instead of lifting both legs off the floor, leave one foot flat on the floor and raise the other so that your heel is 3 to 4 inches off the floor. Then bend at the ankle and move your foot as if you were writing your name or the alphabet in the air. Keep your movements slow and your leg still.

If you have a short name like "Amy," try air writing "Engelbert Humperdinck." That's a mouthful *and* a footful. To make this even more difficult, try raising both legs and writing with both feet at the same time, says exercise physiologist Jennifer Layne.

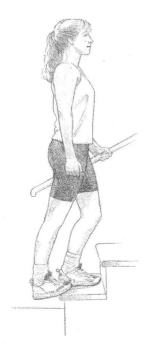

▶ **WHAT IT DOES**

Lengthens your calf muscles

▶ **HOW TO DO IT**

Stand on the bottom step of a staircase and hold on to the railing with one hand to keep your balance. If there is no staircase in your home, you can stand on an aerobic step bench and hold on to a countertop at your side for support. Keep your left foot completely on the step. Move your right foot back so that the ball of your foot is at the edge of the step and your heel hangs off the back. With both knees slightly bent, drop your right heel below the level of the step, then shift your weight so it's over that heel. You should feel a stretch in the back of your lower leg. Hold for 30 seconds, then stretch your left calf.

Key things to remember
• Don't lock knees
• Don't lean forward
• Point toes forward
• Keep feet parallel with each other

The Hips and Butt to Die For

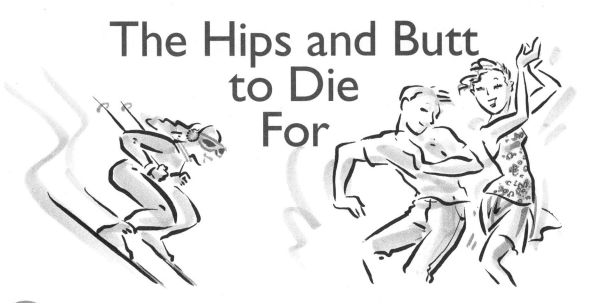

Call it an anatomical irony. The part of our bodies that we sit on all day is potentially one of the strongest areas we have. The major muscle in our buttocks—the gluteus maximus—stretches across the entire tush, and when it's toned, it gives our bottoms their beautiful shapes. The problem is, a layer of fat often hides this muscle, making our rears more rotund than we'd like.

But don't despair. "The muscles along your outer hips and butt are some of the largest muscles in your body, and with the proper exercises, you can dramatically improve the shape of your rear end," says Jennifer Layne, an exercise physiologist at Tufts University in Boston. "Some women avoid exercising this area of their bodies because they're afraid their butts will get bigger," she says. "The truth is, unless you're eating more than you're burning, your butt will not get bigger by exercising it."

Since your hips and butt are your body's powerhouse, making them stronger will help you do daily tasks with greater ease. They're involved in nearly every movement you make, from simply walking to swinging a golf club, Layne says.

Toning will take a two-pronged approach: First, you'll need to do some kind of aerobic exercise, like running or brisk walking, at 60 to 90 percent of your maximum heart rate for 20 to 60 minutes, 3 to 5 days of the week. That's to whittle the layer of fat Layne says. Then, you'll need to tone the muscles in your rear and outer hips to give them definition and shape.

Be patient. Because these muscles are so large, they take longer to firm up than smaller ones. "It could take anywhere from 4 to 6 weeks until you begin to feel stronger and find moving easier. And it will take even longer for you to *see* results," Layne says.

Muscle isn't the only thing you'll build. You'll also build bone and prevent future fractures with these strength-training exercises. "Hip fractures are devastating bone injuries for women as they age," Layne says, "and virtually the only way to build bone in the hip area without medication is with strength training."

The following exercises focus on the three butt muscles—the gluteus maximus, gluteus medius, and gluteus minimus—as well as the muscles that run along the backs of your hips.

THE EXERCISES

Butt Sculptor

▶ **WHAT IT DOES**

Strengthens your buttocks and hip extensors

▶ **IT'S GOOD FOR:**

 cycling

 dancing

 skiing

▶ **GO FOR YOUR GOAL**

Drop a Dress Size: *Two sets of 10 reps on each side, without weights, for 2 to 4 weeks; then two sets of 10 reps on each side with 2- to 3-pound ankle weights*

Shape Up: *Three sets of 8 reps on each side, with 3- to 6-pound ankle weights*

Maintain: *Two to three sets of 8 to 12 reps on each side, with 6- to 10-pound ankle weights*

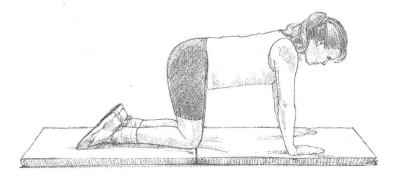

STEP 1: Start on all fours on a mat, with your hands directly under your shoulders and your knees directly under your hips. Keep your back straight and your eyes looking down at the floor. Point your toes and avoid locking your elbows.

Key things to remember
• Don't let stomach sag
• Don't lock elbows
• Keep hips over knees
• Keep shoulders over hands
• Keep neck in line with back

LISTEN TO YOUR BODY

If you feel like you're leaning to one side as you do the butt sculptor, recheck your body alignment. Make sure to keep your butt, back, and neck flat like a table. Your hips and shoulders should be aligned as well. When you lift your leg, push straight up rather than out—pushing your leg out may cause you to twist your hip. Use a slow, smooth movement instead of kicking your leg up.

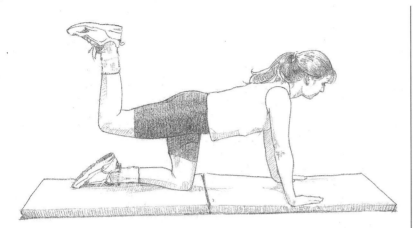

▶ **TAKE IT
TO THE MAX**
To make the butt sculptor a bit more challenging, raise your leg an inch or two higher so that your thigh is slightly above your buttocks in the ending position. Only lift your leg as high as you can without arching your back.

STEP 2: With a slow, smooth movement, lift your right leg straight up while keeping your knee bent at a 90-degree angle. At the end of the move, your right thigh should be parallel to the floor and in line with your right buttock. Hold that position for one count, then lower your leg almost to the starting position for four counts, but don't touch your knee to the floor. Exhale as you lift your leg and inhale as you lower it. After completing your sets with your right leg, repeat with your left.

Key things to remember
- Point toe back
- Keep back flat
- Keep thigh in line with butt
- Bend knee at 90-degree angle

If you feel the effort in your elbows, chances are, you're locking them. Your arms should be straight, just short of locking your elbows.

A strain in your neck means that you're probably arching your head back. Make sure to keep your entire spine straight by lining up your butt, back, and neck. Your head should remain still during the move, with your eyes focused on the floor.

THE EXERCISES

Front Squat

▶ **WHAT IT DOES**
Tones your buttocks, hips, and thighs

▶ **IT'S GOOD FOR:**

 bowling

 golf

 softball

VOL volleyball

▶ **GO FOR YOUR GOAL**

Drop a Dress Size: *Two sets of 10 reps without dumbbells*

Shape Up: *Three sets of 8 reps without dumbbells, until you can squat to where your thighs are parallel to the floor; then three sets of 8 reps with 3- to 5-pound dumbbells*

Maintain: *Two to three sets of 8 to 12 reps without dumbbells, until you can squat to where your thighs are parallel to the floor; then two to three sets of 8 to 12 reps with 5- to 10-pound dumbbells*

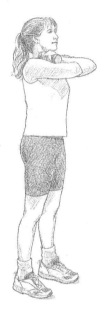

STEP 1: Stand with your feet slightly wider than shoulder-width apart, toes turned slightly outward. If you're using dumbbells, hold one at each shoulder with your arms crossed and your elbows pointing straight ahead. Beginners should do the exercise without weights and may need to hold on to the back of a chair that is secured against a wall for better balance.

Key things to remember
• Stand with good posture
• Keep feet slightly wider than shoulder-width apart
• Point toes out slightly

LISTEN TO YOUR BODY

If you feel like your knees are getting a workout when you do a front squat, you're probably just lowering your body by bending your knees, instead of pushing your buttocks back as you do the move. This common mistake causes your knees to come forward as you squat. To save your knees, aim your buttocks backward and continue to do so while bending your knees. This keeps your knees from coming forward.

If you feel a tug or strain in your lower back, that means that

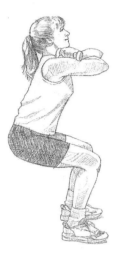

STEP 2: Slowly lower your body into a squat as if you were sitting down in a chair, but don't just drop straight down. Instead, aim your buttocks backward as you lower, keeping your weight balanced back toward your heels. For added safety, place a chair against a wall and aim your buttocks toward the seat. Avoid folding your upper body forward, and lower only as far as you can without moving your knees forward past your toes. Once you've mastered this move, you should be able to lower your body so that your thighs are parallel to the floor. Take four counts to lower into the squat, hold for one count, and then take two counts to come up out of the squat. Don't use momentum to return to the starting position. Instead, contract the muscles in your buttocks and thighs to slowly push yourself up until you're standing straight.

Key things to remember
- Keep upper body erect
- Don't arch back
- Don't lift toes
- Look straight ahead
- Keep thighs parallel to floor
- Don't move knees forward
- Push butt down and back

you're arching your back as you squat, causing your lumbar vertebrae to compress. To fix your form, make sure your back remains straight throughout the exercise.

Check to see if your toes are coming off the floor when you're in the squat position. If they are, that means that you're lowering too far. Lower only as far as you can without lifting your toes.

If you have trouble mastering this move, try doing it in a doorway. Hold on to either side of the doorjamb for balance as you squat. When you do the exercise correctly, your weight should shift backward without your knees moving forward.

▶ **TAKE IT TO THE MAX**
To make the front squat more difficult, make your stance a bit wider and point your toes out a bit more. These minor changes will give your butt and inner thighs a more challenging workout.

Step-Up

  WHAT IT DOES
Tones your gluteus maximus, hamstrings, and quadriceps

▶ **IT'S GOOD FOR:**

CYC cycling

VOL volleyball

▶ **GO FOR YOUR GOAL**

Drop a Dress Size: *Two sets of 10 reps on each side, without dumbbells*

Shape Up: *Three sets of 8 reps on each side with up to 5-pound dumbbells*

Maintain: *Two to three sets of 8 to 12 reps on each side with 5- to 10-pound dumbbells*

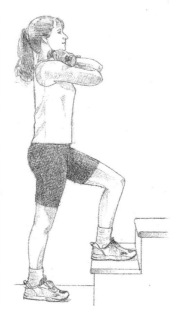

STEP 1: Start with one foot completely on an aerobic step or on the bottom step of a staircase. Plant your other foot on the floor behind you. Make sure the knee of your front leg is directly over your ankle. Beginners should either hold on to the railing lightly for support or cross their arms at their chests. If you're more advanced and using weights for this exercise, hold one dumbbell at each shoulder with your arms crossed and your elbows pointing straight ahead.

Key things to remember
• Keep torso straight
• Keep knee over ankle
• Plant feet firmly

 LISTEN TO YOUR BODY

If you feel discomfort in your front knee when doing a step-up, you're probably letting your knee come forward over your toes. Fix your form by making sure your knee stays directly over your ankle, says exercise physiologist Jennifer Layne.

Another common technique error is to lean forward as you step up. "You want to lift yourself straight up and keep your head and chest lifted," Layne says. "Looking straight ahead rather than

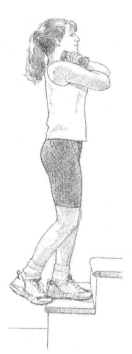

STEP 2: Without pushing off with your back leg, lift your body straight up with your front leg and tap the toes of your back foot on the step. Contract the muscles of your buttocks and the back of your thigh as you lift yourself up. Keep your weight on your front leg during the entire move. Return to the starting position by bringing your foot back down to the floor. Repeat.

Key things to remember
- Look straight ahead
- Keep torso straight
- Keep weight on front foot
- Don't push off with back foot
- Don't allow knee to move forward over your toes

▶ **TAKE IT TO THE MAX**
Once you've mastered the step-up, you can increase the intensity by stepping up two steps instead of one. That may sound like a simple change, but be careful not to try this variation too soon. "You really shouldn't progress to this more advanced version of the exercise until you're able to lift yourself up by using your front leg without any help from your back leg," says exercise physiologist Jennifer Layne. At that point, your back leg should be like deadweight, she adds.

down at your feet can help prevent you from leaning over as well."

If you don't feel the effort in the leg that's on the step, that means that you're pushing off with your back leg. "That's a sign that you're not strong enough to use only your front leg to lift yourself up," Layne says. In that case, you should use a lower step, like an aerobics step. You should also do the exercise without dumbbells until you're able to lift yourself up entirely with your front leg, without pushing off with your back leg.

THE EXERCISES

Grand Plié Second Position

▶ **WHAT IT DOES**
Strengthens your gluteus muscles and hip extensors

▶ **GO FOR YOUR GOAL**
Drop a Dress Size: *8 to 10 reps*
Shape Up: *10 to 16 reps*
Maintain: *16 to 18 reps*

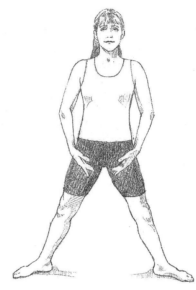

STEP 1: Begin in ballet second position, with your heels 2 to 2½ feet apart and your toes pointed to 2 and 10 o'clock. Your arms should be rounded, with your fingertips curving slightly toward each other. Your shoulders should be back. If you need to, you can hold on to the back of a chair for balance.

Key things to remember
• Don't lock knees
• Keep torso straight
• Press shoulders down

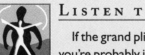

LISTEN TO YOUR BODY

If the grand plié second position seems quite easy, you're probably just plopping yourself down and standing back up. This move is not merely a knee bend, but rather an exercise that requires a lot of internal resistance. When you do a plié, you always need to create a sense of pulling in the opposite direction from where you're going. This internal resistance gives you better balance and posture and brings more muscles into the exercise.

STEP 2: Before you bend your knees, pull upward in your torso and hips to maintain proper alignment and better muscular control. Then start the downward move from your hips, not just from your knees. Lower into the plié position, maintaining control of your torso muscles as if you were wearing a corset. As you lower 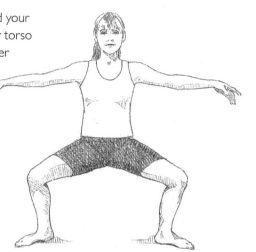 into the plié, raise your straightened arms out to your sides, keeping your hands below shoulder level. While in the plié, press your heels down into the floor and don't let your knees roll forward. Keep your buttocks and abs flexed throughout the move. Return to the starting position by contracting your inner-thigh and buttocks muscles and pressing your heels down as you straighten your legs. Repeat.

Key things to remember
- Tighten abs
- Don't let knees rotate forward
- Press heels down

▶ **TAKE IT TO THE MAX**
To make the grand plié second position even more challenging, go even lower on the downward move and do the entire exercise more slowly, as if you are moving in slow motion. "The muscles that you're working in this move are large and take a long time to fatigue," says certified personal trainer Karen Andes. "Going slowly keeps those muscles in constant resistance, so you work them with greater intensity."

When you move down into the plié, imagine that your upper body has pulleys attached to it that are pulling you up as you move down. When you return from the plié to the starting position, create resistance by pressing down as you lift your body up.

It may also help to imagine that your legs don't end at your hips, but instead go all of the way up to under your armpits. As you go up, pretend that you're pulling on a pair of support hose all the way up to your armpits.

THE EXERCISES

Arabesque Raise

▶ **WHAT IT DOES**
Tones your glutes, hip extensors, and hamstrings

▶ **GO FOR YOUR GOAL**
Drop a Dress Size: *8 to 12 reps*
Shape Up: *12 to 16 reps*
Maintain: *16 to 20 reps*

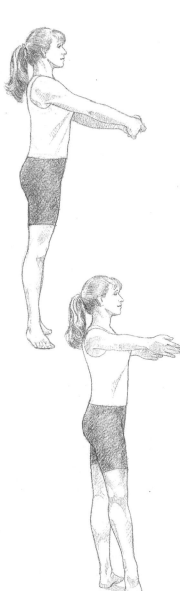

STEP 1: Begin in ballet first position, with your toes turned to 2 and 10 o'clock and with proper posture. Your thighs, calves, and heels should touch. Extend and round your arms slightly below your chest as if you're holding a beach ball. Keep your shoulders back and your abs and buttocks taut. If necessary, hold on to the back of a chair for balance.

Key things to remember
• Tighten abs
• Squeeze buttocks
• Maintain proper posture
• Round arms below chest
• Stand with heels together

STEP 2: Sweep your right leg out to the side, flex your thigh and calf, and point your right toes. Bend your left knee slightly so that it is not locked. Raise your arms to your chest and open them as if you're about to give someone a hug.

Key things to remember
• Open arms
• Point toes
• Flex thigh and calf

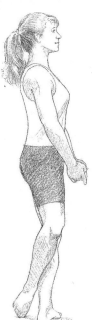

STEP 3: Transfer your weight to your left leg as you lift your right leg and bend your right knee behind you. Rest your right calf against your left calf so that your right knee points out to the side and your right toes remain pointed. Keeping your arms rounded, lower them and bring your hands closer together in front of your upper thighs.

Key things to remember
- Don't lock knee of supporting leg
- Round arms in front of thighs
- Point knee out to side
- Point toes

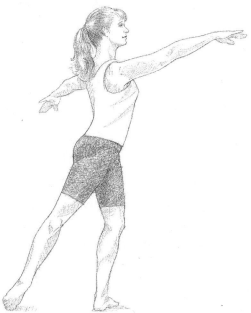

STEP 4: While balancing your weight on your left leg, straighten and raise your right leg slightly behind you. Keep your right hip facing forward, and keep your right knee pointing out to the side. Place your arms in the arabesque position, with your right hand just above shoulder level and your left hand extended out to the side.

Key things to remember
- Lift leg slightly off floor
- Keep knee bent slightly
- Raise hand in line with nose
- Keep torso straight
- Don't turn hip out

(continued)

THE EXERCISES

Arabesque Raise—Continued

▶ **TAKE IT
TO THE MAX**
The advanced exerciser
can make the arabesque
raise more difficult just by
doing repetitions be-
tween the third, fourth,
and fifth steps. "They're
the hardest parts of the
move, so repeating those
three steps will give you
the best workout," says
certified personal trainer
Karen Andes.

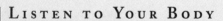

STEP 5: Reach
back with your right leg as
you raise it farther off the floor.
An experienced ballerina would
keep her torso in a straight line,
but you may have to incline your
torso forward about 3 inches if this
position bothers your lower back.
Keep your arms in the arabesque position. Hold for at least one count.
Then lower your arms and back leg
into the starting position and repeat.

Key things to remember
• Keep torso straight or slightly for-
ward
• Raise leg higher off floor
• Point toe

LISTEN TO YOUR BODY

If you feel a strain in your lower back when you do the arabesque raise, you're
not adequately holding in your torso with your abdominal muscles. Remember to
pull in your abs as you do the move. Doing so will not only prevent lower-back
pain, but it will also help you maintain proper posture.

If you feel effort in your supporting knee, check your form to make sure your knee is not
locked and your foot is not turned out too far. Your right toes should point to 2 o'clock and
your left toes to 10 o'clock.

THE STRETCHES

Buttocks Stretch

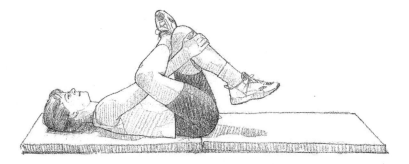

▶ WHAT IT DOES
Lengthens your three gluteus muscles

▶ HOW TO DO IT
Lie flat on your back with your knees bent and your feet flat on the floor. Place your right ankle on your left knee so that your right knee points out to your right side. The small of your back should be pressed against the floor, and the bottom of your buttocks should tilt upward slightly. Reach around and place both hands on the shin of your left leg just below your knee, and gently pull your leg in toward your chest. You should feel the stretch in your buttocks and in the outer thigh of your right leg. Hold for 30 seconds, then stretch the other side.

Key things to remember
• Point knee outward
• Keep head on floor
• Pull leg toward chest

THE STRETCHES

Hip Stretch

▶ **DESKTOP TRAINER**

Wall Sit

Stand with your back and feet against a wall, feet about hip-width apart. Then slowly slide your back down the wall while walking your feet out until it's as if you're sitting in a chair. Stay in that position for a count of 5 to 10 seconds, then slide back up. Repeat five times. As you become stronger, hold the position longer.

Here are a few things to watch out for. Keep your back straight and pressed against the wall throughout the move. Lower only to where your thighs are parallel to the floor; don't slide farther down than that. In addition, don't let your knees go beyond your toes. Finally, wear shoes with some grip on the soles so that your feet don't slip out from under you, says exercise physiologist Jennifer Layne.

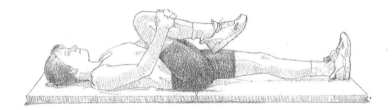

▶ **WHAT IT DOES**

Increases flexibility in your hip extensors and gluteus maximus

▶ **HOW TO DO IT**

Lie on your back with your lower back pressed against the floor and your legs straight. Bend your right knee and bring it toward your chest. Interlace your hands on the shin of your right leg, just below your knee, and gently pull your right thigh toward your chest. Keep your left leg straight. Your hips should be even and flat on the floor. Hold for 30 seconds and then stretch your left leg.

Key things to remember
- Don't lift straight leg off floor
- Point toes up
- Look straight up

The Belly Vanishing Act

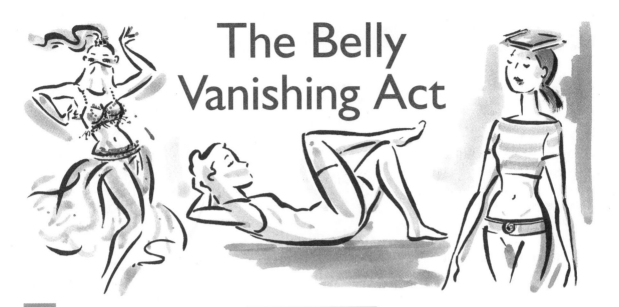

The most difficult tricks are usually the best. Ask any magician.

Maybe that's why a trim waistline is so impressive. Getting rid of a belly is not easy.

Toning, by itself, won't do it. The reason: Whittling away your waist has a lot more to do with shedding fat than with building muscle. "Your abdominal muscles could be strong and nicely developed, but if they're under a layer of fat, you're not going to see them," says Jennifer Layne, an exercise physiologist at Tufts University in Boston.

So if losing extra pounds around your middle is a top priority, a minimum of 20 minutes of aerobic exercise at least three times a week is what you need. So is eating a healthy, low-fat diet. Then, polish your look by adding the toning exercises that follow.

These exercises target all of your abdominal muscles, from the external and internal obliques, which stretch over your rib cage along your sides, to the rectus abdominis, which run vertically from your chest to your pelvis. They also work the transversus abdominis, which run across your midsection (underneath the other abdom-inal muscles) and hold in your stomach, like a natural girdle.

Developing these muscles will make your middle firmer. And as your abs become stronger, your posture will improve, making you appear thinner, Layne says. Having strong abdominal muscles also makes everything from bending down to lifting and twisting easier, not to mention safer.

"Your abdomen, along with your lower back, forms what is really the core of your body," Layne says. That's where your center of gravity is; and it's essentially where almost all of your movement comes from. For that reason, your core is really the most important area in your body to strengthen. "If you tone just your arms and legs and then lift something heavy because you feel stronger, you're likely to hurt yourself," she explains, "because it's actually your core—not your limbs—that bears the brunt of the weight you're lifting."

So for your health and your figure, check out the following ab exercises. If you do them regularly, along with aerobic exercises, and maintain a healthy diet, you're bound to have a firmer, flatter belly in about 2 months. Abracadabra.

THE EXERCISES

Abdominal Crunch

▶ **WHAT IT DOES**
Strengthens all of your
abdominal muscles

▶ **IT'S GOOD FOR:**
All sports

▶ **GO FOR YOUR GOAL**

Drop a Dress Size: *Two
sets of 10 reps*

Shape Up: *Three sets of
8 reps*

Maintain: *Two to three
sets of 8 to 12 reps*

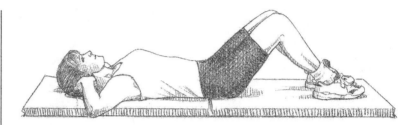

STEP 1: Lie face-up on a mat with your knees bent and your feet flat on the
floor. Place your feet about hip-width apart. Place your fingertips behind your
ears to gently support your head and to keep your head and neck in proper
alignment. Keep your elbows as close to the floor as possible. Your lower
back should be flat against the floor, not arching. This is the starting position.

Key things to remember
• Keep feet flat, about hip-width apart
• Hold fingertips behind ears
• Keep elbows close to floor
• Press lower back against floor

LISTEN TO YOUR BODY

Check to make sure you're not making two
common mistakes when you do abdominal crunches.
First, are you holding your breath? "People often hold
their breath when they do abdominal work," says exercise physiologist Jennifer Layne. Make sure you're exhaling as you lift your
torso and inhaling as you lower.

Another common error is doing the move too fast. You won't be
giving your abs a real workout if you use momentum to bounce up
and down off the floor, Layne says. Make sure you're crunching in a
slow, controlled movement. It may help to count 2 full seconds
(one-Mississippi, two-Mississippi) as you lift and lower.

If you don't feel the effort in your abdomen, that means you're

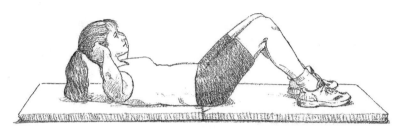

STEP 2: Contract the muscles in your abdomen and slowly lift your torso so that your shoulder blades come off the floor. Beginners may be able to come up only 1 to 2 inches. Support your head with your hands as you come up, but avoid pulling your head forward. Keep your eyes focused on the ceiling. Take two counts to lift your torso, hold for one count, and then lower your torso back to the starting position for two counts. Exhale as you lift and inhale as you lower. Repeat.

Key things to remember
• Support head
• Lift shoulder blades off floor
• Look up at ceiling
• Press lower back against floor
• Hold elbows out to sides

using your arms to pull your head and torso up off the floor, Layne says. Focus on contracting your abs to bring your body up. Discomfort in your neck is another sign that you're probably pulling your head off the floor with your arms, she says. To fix your form, concentrate on gently supporting your head with your fingertips and using your abs to lift yourself off the floor. It helps to keep your elbows out to your sides, rather than bringing them forward.

You could also feel discomfort in your neck if you're coming up higher than your abs are strong enough to lift you. "The key is to really listen to your body and work through your own range of motion, rather than coming up as high as you think you should," Layne explains. "Come up just a few inches and stop before you feel that discomfort in your neck, because once you feel the discomfort, you've come up too far."

▶ **TAKE IT TO THE MAX**
You can give your abs a more challenging workout if you do abdominal crunches with your legs raised off the floor. Start with your legs straight up in the air so that your trunk and torso form an L. Cross your feet at your ankles, and be careful not to lock your knees. Stay in this position as you lift your torso off the floor with your abs. "You can progress to this more advanced position after you have mastered the regular abdominal crunch and can comfortably lift your shoulder blades off the floor with each repetition," says exercise physiologist Jennifer Layne.

THE EXERCISES

Abdominal Crunch with Rotation

▶ **WHAT IT DOES**
Works all of your ab
muscles

▶ **IT'S GOOD FOR:**

 dancing

 golf

 skiing

 tennis

 volleyball

▶ **GO FOR YOUR GOAL**

Drop a Dress Size: *Two
sets of 10 reps on each side*

Shape Up: *Three sets of
8 reps on each side*

Maintain: *Two to three
sets of 8 to 12 reps on
each side*

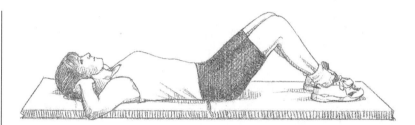

STEP 1: Lie face-up on a mat with your knees bent and your feet flat on
the floor. Place your feet about hip-width apart. Place your fingertips behind your ears to gently support your head and to keep your head and
neck in proper alignment. Keep your elbows as close to the floor as possible. Your lower back should be flat against the floor, not arching. This is
the starting position.

Key things to remember
• Keep feet flat, about hip-width apart
• Hold fingertips behind ears
• Keep elbows close to floor
• Press lower back against floor

LISTEN TO YOUR BODY

If your elbows come forward as you come off the
floor during a crunch with rotation, that means you're
moving your arms toward your knee instead of your
shoulder to your knee, and you're probably not rotating your torso
the way that you should, says exercise physiologist Jennifer Layne.
Here's how to fix your form. As you come up, concentrate on rotating your torso from the waist so your shoulder, not your elbow,
goes in the direction of your opposite knee, Layne suggests. Keep
your elbows pointed out to your sides and concentrate on using
only your fingertips to support your head.

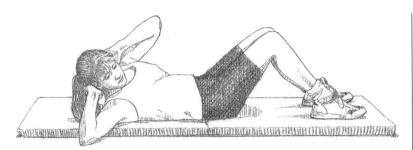

STEP 2: Contract the muscles in your abdomen and slowly lift your torso so that your shoulder blades come off the floor. As you come up, gently rotate your torso from the waist so that your left shoulder goes toward your right knee. Support your head with your hands, but avoid pulling your head forward. Take two counts to lift and rotate your torso, hold for one count, and then rotate and lower your torso back to the starting position for two counts. On your next repetition, rotate your torso so that your right shoulder goes toward your left knee. Continue alternating sides with each repetition.

Key things to remember
- Support head
- Lift shoulder blades off floor
- Press lower back against floor
- Hold elbows back
- Rotate shoulder toward opposite knee
- Move from the waist

▶ **TAKE IT TO THE MAX**
Once you have the crunch with rotation down pat, you can make it more difficult by first coming straight up off the floor for one count as if you are doing a regular abdominal crunch without rotation. Once your torso is off the floor, rotate your shoulder toward the opposite knee for one count. Take two counts to lower back to the floor: First, rotate so your torso is no longer twisted. Then lower straight down to the floor as if you were coming out of the regular abdominal crunch.

If you feel strain or discomfort in your side or back, you may be twisting too much or doing the move too quickly. Remember, this is a slow, controlled movement. Feeling strain in your back or side could also mean that you're not quite ready for this exercise. "The crunch with rotation is a more advanced exercise. It should only be attempted by those who can completely lift their shoulder blades off the floor when doing an abdominal crunch without rotation," Layne says.

Once you *are* ready for this move, strive to use the best technique that you possibly can, Layne says. Don't be concerned if you are not able to rotate as far as the fitness professionals you may have seen on TV or in exercise videos, she adds.

Pelvic Tilt

▶ **WHAT IT DOES**
Targets all of your abdominal muscles

▶ **IT'S GOOD FOR:**

 dancing

 skiing

▶ **GO FOR YOUR GOAL**

Drop a Dress Size: *Two sets of 10 reps*

Shape Up: *Three sets of 8 reps*

Maintain: *Two to three sets of 8 to 12 reps*

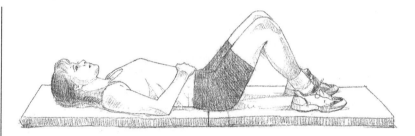

STEP 1: To start, lie face-up on a mat with your knees bent and your feet flat on the floor. Your feet should be about hip-width apart. Place one hand on your stomach so you'll be able to feel your abs contracting when you do the move.

Key things to remember
• Keep feet flat, about hip-width apart
• Put hand on stomach

LISTEN TO YOUR BODY

If you feel the effort in the front of your thighs when you do a pelvis tilt, that means you're using your legs to lift your buttocks up instead of lifting them by contracting your abs, says exercise physiologist Jennifer Layne. To fix your form, keep your thighs still and relaxed when you do this

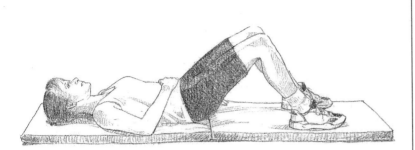

STEP 2: While pressing the small of your back against the floor, contract your abdominal muscles and use them to tilt your pelvis toward your shoulders. Press your abs downward slightly as you tilt. Your pelvis and the bottom of your buttocks should come slightly off the floor. You should not be lifting straight up, but rather curling the bottom of your buttocks, the tail of your spine, and your hips toward your shoulders. The movement is very small—you may tilt up only about 3 inches. The hand on your stomach should feel your abdomen pressing down toward the floor as you tilt your pelvis and lower butt. Take two counts to contract your abs and tilt, hold for one count, and lower for two. Exhale as you tilt, and inhale as you return to the starting position.

Key things to remember

• Press abdomen down
• Tilt hips up and back toward shoulders
• Press lower back against floor

move. It may help to think of the movement as a tilt rather than a lift. And remember that only the lower part of your butt actually comes off the floor, at least in the beginning. "As you become stronger, you'll be able to tilt higher so that more of your butt comes up," Layne says.

▶ **TAKE IT
TO THE MAX**

Once you've mastered the pelvic tilt, you can make it more difficult by putting your feet up on an aerobic step. Place your heels on the edge of the step, with your feet pointing straight up. Your legs should be bent at an angle that's halfway between 90 degrees and straight legs. Perform the move, making sure that you do not move your feet or lower legs. Press your heels down, but don't rock your toes forward. This variation works your butt and hamstrings as well as your abs. As you become stronger, you'll be able to tilt your butt completely up and off the floor.

You can make this move even more challenging by keeping just one leg on the step. Cross your right leg over your left by resting your right ankle just below your left knee. Then contract and press your abs down as you tilt your lower butt and pelvis toward your shoulders. Repeat the move with your right foot on the step.

THE EXERCISES

Reverse Curl

▶ **WHAT IT DOES**
Strengthens all of your abdominal muscles

▶ **IT'S GOOD FOR:**

 dancing

 volleyball

▶ **GO FOR YOUR GOAL**

Drop a Dress Size: *Two sets of 10 reps*

Shape Up: *Three sets of 8 reps*

Maintain: *Two to three sets of 8 to 12 reps*

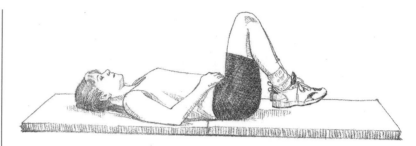

STEP 1: To start, lie face-up on a mat with one arm on your stomach and one arm down at your side. Keeping your lower back pressed against the floor, raise your legs off the mat so that your thighs form a right angle with your upper body. Your legs should be together and bent at the knees, with your lower legs relaxed and your calves touching the backs of your thighs. Place one hand on your stomach so you can feel your abs contracting when you do the move.

Key things to remember
• Press lower back against floor
• Keep thighs and body at right angle
• Relax lower legs
• Put hand on stomach

LISTEN TO YOUR BODY

The reverse curl is an advanced exercise for the fitter woman. "This is the next step after you've mastered the pelvic tilt, which is a similar but smaller movement," explains exercise physiologist Jennifer Layne.

If you are ready for the reverse curl, keep these tips in mind: The most common mistake that women make when they do this exercise is to use momentum, rather than their abdominal muscles, to bring their knees toward their chests. "Just rocking your lower body

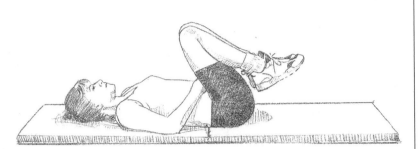

STEP 2: Contract your abs, moving from your hips, tilting your pelvis up and back, and slowly bring your knees toward your chest. Bring your knees in as far as you comfortably can without rocking your body. (That may be only a few inches.) Take two counts to bring your knees to your chest, hold for one count, and then return to the starting position for two counts by moving your knees away from your chest. Exhale as you bring your knees toward your chest, and inhale as you return to the starting position. Repeat.

Key things to remember
- Bring knees toward chest
- Contract abs
- Press lower back against floor
- Don't rock

▶ **TAKE IT TO THE MAX**

You can give your abs a more challenging workout by doing the reverse curl with your legs raised up in the air, rather than bent at the knees, says exercise physiologist Jennifer Layne. Your legs should be together with your feet crossed at your ankles. Just make sure your knees are slightly bent and back so that your thighs are perpendicular to the floor, she cautions. Contract your abs and bring your legs toward your chest as far as you comfortably can without rocking your body. Hold for one count, then return to the starting position. Repeat.

toward your chest isn't going to do anything for your abs," Layne explains. The key to doing this move correctly is to squeeze your abs while bringing your knees in with a slow, controlled movement. "If your knees only come a few inches toward your chest, that's okay. But if you bring your knees all the way to your chest, you're probably rocking."

Another thing to watch out for: Make sure you don't hold your breath, Layne says. You should exhale as you bring your knees toward your chest and inhale as you return to the starting position.

THE EXERCISES

Ab Stabilizer

▶ **WHAT IT DOES**
Develops your rectus and transversus abdominis muscles

▶ **IT'S GOOD FOR:**
All sports

▶ **GO FOR YOUR GOAL**
Drop a Dress Size: *8 to 10 reps*
Shape Up: *10 to 16 reps*
Maintain: *16 to 20 reps*

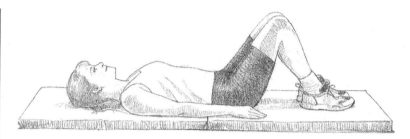

STEP 1: Lie face-up on a mat, with your arms straight by your sides. Bend your knees so that your feet are flat on the floor, about hip-width apart. This is the starting position.

Key things to remember
• Keep feet flat, hip-width apart
• Lay arms at sides

LISTEN TO YOUR BODY

The key to doing the ab stabilizer correctly is to really cave in your abdomen. "It should feel as if your belly button is being pulled down through your stomach to your spine," says certified personal trainer Karen Andes.

If you don't pull your abs in, you may feel some strain in your back, Andes says. It's okay to press your lower back against the floor if it doesn't cause tension in your neck and shoulders or collapse your abdominal muscles. You can also maintain a slight natural curve in your lower back. Whatever style of this exercise you choose, don't change it.

Another form fine point: The top of your head should face up toward the ceiling, and your neck should feel as if it's lengthened, Andes says. If you have trouble keeping your head and neck in this position, you can do the exercise with your head down on the floor.

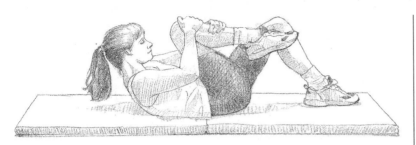

STEP 2: Lift your head and bring your right knee toward your chest, pointing your toes. Hold your right leg in place by grasping your leg at your knee and shin. Your chin should be tucked but not touching your chest, as if you're holding an orange under it.

Key things to remember
- Hold shin parallel with floor
- Point toes
- Tuck chin

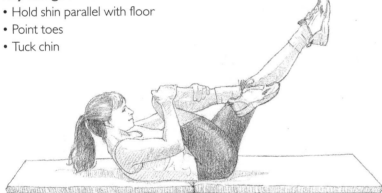

STEP 3: Exhale as you pull in your abs and raise your straightened left leg so that it's at about a 45-degree angle to the floor. As you lift your leg, try to keep your head and upper body still. Inhale. For an easier version, you can raise your leg with your knee bent so that your leg is vertical and in the shape of an L.

Key things to remember
- Point toes
- Keep head still
- Press lower back against floor
- Pull abs downward
- Hold leg straight, at 45-degree angle to floor

(continued)

▶ **TAKE IT
TO THE MAX**
To make the ab stabilizer even more challenging, keep your extended leg closer to the floor. "The closer that leg is to the floor, the harder your abs have to work," says certified personal trainer Karen Andes.

Ab Stabilizer—Continued

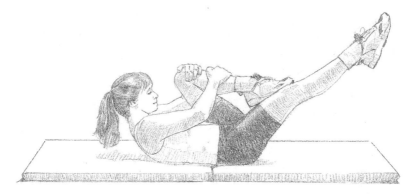

STEP 4: Contract your abs and keep your head and torso still as you take one or two counts to switch the positions of your legs. After the switch, your right leg should be extended at about a 45-degree angle to the floor, and your left leg should be pulled toward your chest. Make sure your shoulders are lifted off the floor, but that they're not hunched up or rounded forward. Hold the position for two counts, then switch the position of your legs again. Count each leg switch as a repetition. Beginners should do this move slowly, taking about four counts for every leg switch. Once you've mastered the move, you can take two counts to switch and hold.

Key things to remember
- Contract abs
- Press lower back against floor
- Keep rest of body still
- Switch position of legs
- Don't hunch or round shoulders

Side Bend

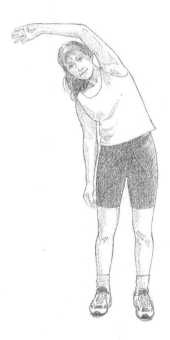

▶ **WHAT IT DOES**
Stretches your oblique muscles

▶ **HOW TO DO IT**
Start by standing up straight with your arms down at your sides. Your feet should be about hip-width apart, with your toes pointing forward. Raise your left arm straight up with a slight bend at the elbow as if you were raising your hand to ask a question at a meeting. Your right arm should remain down at your side. Slowly bend at your waist over your right side. Make sure your torso does not fold forward. Hold this position for 30 seconds. Then stand up straight before bending at your waist over your left side and holding for 30 seconds.

Key things to remember
• Bend to side, not forward
• Keep feet hip-width apart, toes pointing forward
• Keep arm slightly bent

▶ **DESKTOP TRAINER**

Seated Trunk Twist

This exercise will stretch your obliques, says exercise physiologist Jennifer Layne. It can also help relieve back tension for those who spend long periods of time seated in a chair.

Sit off the right side of your chair so that your body and legs face sideways and the edge of the seat is at the bend in your knees. Your feet should be flat on the floor, about hip-width apart. Slowly rotate your torso, from your waist up, as far toward the right as you comfortably can. Your head and shoulders should move with your body. Hold on to the back of the chair to maintain the stretch for 30 seconds, making sure not to hold your breath. Then return to the starting position. Repeat three times, then sit off the left side of the chair and rotate to the left.

Today, Tania Sobrino is a tall, fit, 31-year-old paralegal who is completing her journalism degree at Rutgers University in New Brunswick, New Jersey, and working on her certification to become a personal trainer. But she used to be overweight, suffering from low self-esteem, and struggling with a borderline eating disorder. How did she make such a big change? Here's her story.

My weight had been a struggle for me my entire life. I was never what you'd call obese, but I was always carrying around an extra 20 to 30 pounds. When I was 15, I saw the movie *Flashdance*, and that got me working out a little, but it was nothing lasting. When I was 19, I had a boyfriend who constantly criticized me about my weight. What I ended up doing in my teens and early twenties was all the wrong things.

I dieted. I binged. I used diet pills. I got into the aerobics craze, but I'd force myself to perform hours of pure cardio work—then I'd go home and eat a bag of chocolate chip cookies.

One thing that I tried really did "work." I semi-starved myself, eating next to nothing for 6 weeks. Sure enough, those 30 pounds went away, though I had no idea how much harm I was doing to my body. What I did know is that I looked pale and weak, with no muscle tone at all. And I felt like hell.

Then, about 4 years ago, I had an experience that changed my life. My great-aunt went through a grueling recovery from hip-replacement surgery. When I looked at her, I realized that she was what I had always thought was the only thing that I wanted to be—thin. But, of course, she had never exercised a day in her life, so her muscles were very weak with age. What's more, her physical therapist mentioned that if she had strength trained earlier in life, she could have avoided the osteoporosis that made the surgery necessary.

All of this was a revelation to me. For one thing, I had never known that strength training was good for your bones. But more important, I realized right then and there that thin doesn't necessarily mean healthy. I did not want to go through what my aunt was going through. And I did not want to live the rest of my life being weak and dependent. At that moment, I knew that strength training would help me.

Of course, I still included aerobic exercise in my routine, and I also made a commitment to eat more healthfully. But my weight training really improved my resting metabolic rate, which helped me burn calories more efficiently. I saw dramatic changes in my body very quickly. I dropped three dress sizes and 27 pounds in about 7 months. The results were amazing!

Now, for the first time in my life, I am honestly happy with my body. I no longer hide under long black dresses. With my newfound love of strength training and with the constant, loving support of my husband, I've overcome my eating disorder and made peace with my body—and myself.

I'm so grateful for what weight training has done for me that I'm planning on becoming a personal trainer so I can help others change their lives the right way. I guess that some women find it hard to believe that their lives can change through exercise alone. But I know it's true, because I'm living proof.

How to Bust with Pride

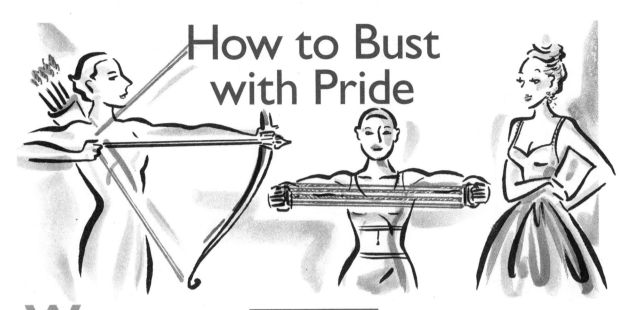

When we were 13 years old, we wore the tightest shirts and sweaters that our allowances could buy to show off our budding breasts—much to our fathers' chagrin. But something happened between our 13th and 35th birthdays. Gravity had taken hold.

It seems that there are few ways to give our bustlines a makeover, short of having surgery, stocking up on Wonderbras, or moving to the moon (where gravity doesn't pull down so hard). In fact, more than 130,000 women in the United States opted for breast-implant surgery last year, shelling out about $3,000 per operation to enhance the size and shape of their breasts.

There is another way, and it's a lot kinder to your pocketbook. Lifting weights can actually help you defy gravity without the risks of surgery. Here's how.

Breast tissue is basically nothing more than fat, connective tissue, and mammary glands, says Jennifer Layne, an exercise physiologist at Tufts University in Boston. Underneath your breasts are two muscles called the pectoralis major and minor. "When they're toned, they act like an underwire of muscle that gives your breasts a bit of a lift," Layne says. Granted, the results won't be as dramatic as surgery, she says, and they'll vary depending on your cup size.

Smaller-chested women will not only get a lift but they'll also appear bigger. "You'll have the appearance of larger breasts because the breast tissue will be lifted and supported by the well-defined muscles beneath it," Layne explains. "You won't actually increase the size of your breasts."

Larger-busted women will see the best results if they lose weight slowly and tone their chest muscles, Layne says. Because breasts are mostly fat, they often shrink in size when you shed a few pounds. And the smaller your breasts, the perkier they'll appear when the muscles underneath are developed.

You'll start to see changes in your bustline after doing these exercises for 4 to 6 weeks. Developed chest muscles come in handy in other ways as well. Whether you're working out on a rowing machine or doing some shoveling in your garden, strong pectoralis muscles make downward and forward pushing movements easier. Strong chest muscles also help to stabilize your shoulders and your improve posture.

Chest Press

▶ **WHAT IT DOES**
Tones your pectoralis major and minor

▶ **IT'S GOOD FOR:**
All sports

▶ **GO FOR YOUR GOAL**

Drop a Dress Size: *Two sets of 10 reps with 2- to 5-pound dumbbells*

Shape Up: *Three sets of 8 reps with 5- to 10-pound dumbbells*

Maintain: *Two to three sets of 8 to 12 reps with 10- to 15-pound dumbbells*

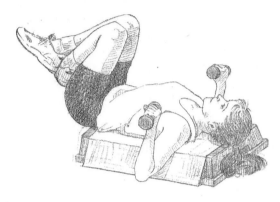

STEP 1: Place a towel on an aerobic step. Lie face-up so that your head, back, and buttocks are all on the step. Bring your thighs toward your chest, with your feet crossed at the ankles. This position helps keep the small of your back pressed against the step. Maintain this position throughout the exercise to protect your lower back. Start with a dumbbell in each hand, with your palms facing forward and your knuckles facing up. Hold the dumbbells out to the sides of your mid-chest and above the level of your body, making sure to keep your wrists straight and in line with your hands. Your elbows should be just below the level of the step and should point down to the floor. Your forearms should be straight up and down and parallel to each other, with your wrists and elbows in a straight line.

Key things to remember
• Raise thighs toward chest
• Face palms forward
• Face knuckles up
• Hold wrists straight
• Hold dumbbells out to sides of mid-chest, above body level
• Keep elbows below step-level, pointing down
• Align wrists with elbows

STEP 2: Keeping the small of your back against the step, press the dumbbells straight up so that your arms are fully extended, with your wrists, elbows, and shoulders in a straight line. Make sure not to lock your elbows. Exhale as you lift the dumb- bells for two counts. Hold for one count at the end of the lift. Then inhale as you take four counts to lower the dumbbells back to the starting position.

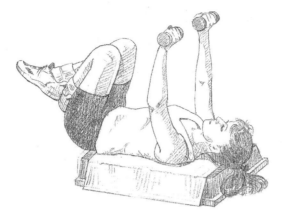

Key things to remember
• Keep wrists straight
• Align wrists, elbows, and shoulders
• Don't lock elbows
• Press lower back against step

▶ **TAKE IT TO THE MAX**
You can make the chest press a bit more difficult by contracting your chest muscles through a greater range of motion, says ex- ercise physiologist Jennifer Layne. To do that, bring your shoulders blades apart slightly to fully flex your chest muscles as you lift the dumbbells. Then bring your shoulder blades back together as you lower the dumbbells. It's a very small move- ment, maybe only an inch, but you will feel the differ- ence, Layne says.

LISTEN TO YOUR BODY

Here are some tips to help you get the most out of the chest press. First, avoid bringing the dumbbells below chest level in the starting position, cautions exercise physiologist Jennifer Layne. Second, make sure you press both dumbbells up at the same pace. Third, you also need to press your back against the step so that you don't arch it to help you lift. Finally, you should check that you bring the dumbbells down so they're just out to the sides of the middle of your chest after each repetition. "Sometimes beginners let the dumb- bells drift up toward their necks," Layne says.

One important safety consideration with this exercise is getting into position with the dumb- bells, especially if you exercise alone. Hold one dumbbell in each hand, close to your body, says Layne. Then sit on the step and roll back into position, keeping the weights close to you. To get up from the step when you're done, put one dumbbell down on the floor at your side, put the other down at your other side, and then roll up from the step.

THE EXERCISES

Chest Fly

▶ **WHAT IT DOES**
Strengthens your pectoralis major and minor

▶ **IT'S GOOD FOR:**

GLF golf

SB softball

TEN tennis

▶ **GO FOR YOUR GOAL**

Drop a Dress Size: *Two sets of 10 reps with 2- to 5-pound dumbbells*

Shape Up: *Three sets of 8 reps with 5- to 8-pound dumbbells*

Maintain: *Two to three sets of 8 to 12 reps with 8- to 12-pound dumbbells*

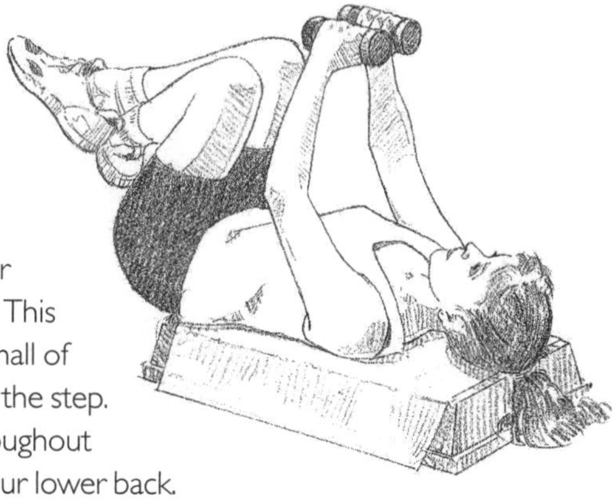

STEP 1: Place a towel on an aerobic step. Lie face-up so that your head, back, and buttocks are all on the step. Bring your thighs toward your chest, with your feet crossed at the ankles. This position helps keep the small of your back pressed against the step. Maintain this position throughout the exercise to protect your lower back. Start with a dumbbell in each hand. Extend your arms straight up above your mid-chest so that your palms face each other and the dumbbells are close together. Your elbows should be bent slightly out to the sides, as if you were hugging a tree. Keep your wrists straight and in line with your hands.

Key things to remember
• Press lower back against step
• Raise thighs toward chest
• Extend arms above mid-chest
• Keep wrists straight
• Bend elbows slightly out to sides

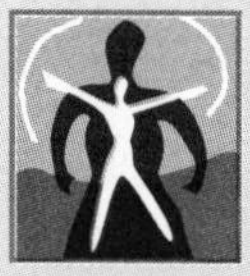

LISTEN TO YOUR BODY

The movement for the chest fly comes from your chest and your upper arms, says exercise physiologist Jennifer Layne. One key element to this move is to maintain the same bend in your elbow, she says. "Make sure not to straighten your arms by unbending your elbows as you lower the weights, and don't let the dumbbells drop below chest level at the bottom of the move," she says.

STEP 2: Inhale as you move the dumbbells out and down in a wide arc for four counts. Lead the way down with your elbows, making sure to maintain the same bend in them from start to finish. At the end of the move, your elbows should point down and should be below the level of the step. The dumbbells should be in line with your mid-chest and should not drop below shoulder level. Hold this position for one count. Then exhale as you take two counts to lift the dumbbells back to the starting position.

Key things to remember
- Point elbows down
- Lower elbows to just below level of step
- Hold dumbbells mid-chest
- Don't curl wrists
- Press lower back against step
- Keep elbows slightly bent

▶ **TAKE IT TO THE MAX**

The technique used to make the chest press more challenging applies here as well. To contract your chest muscles through a greater range of motion, squeeze your shoulder blades together slightly when your arms are in the down position. Then bring your shoulders blades apart slightly to contract your chest muscles as you lift the dumbbells.

As with the chest press, keep the small of your back against the step during the exercise, and be careful when getting in and out of position with the weights. Make sure to hold one dumbbell in each hand, keeping them close to your body as you sit on the step and roll back into position. To get up from the step when you're done, Layne advises, put the dumbbells down on the floor at your sides, one at a time, and then roll up from the step.

Modified Pushup

▶ **WHAT IT DOES**
Tones your chest muscles

▶ **IT'S GOOD FOR:**

◆DAN▶ dancing

◆TEN▶ tennis

◆VOL▶ volleyball

▶ **GO FOR YOUR GOAL**
Drop a Dress Size: *2 reps*
Shape Up: *4 reps*
Maintain: *6 reps*

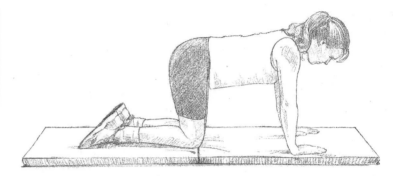

STEP 1: To start, kneel on all fours on a mat, with your knees and feet hip-width apart. Place your hands directly under your shoulders and your knees directly under your hips. Keep your back flat and look down at the floor so that your neck is in line with your spine.

Key things to remember
• Keep back flat
• Align neck with spine
• Align hands with shoulders
• Align knees with hips

LISTEN TO YOUR BODY

When you're in the downward-facing-dog pose during the modified pushup, make sure your heels are slightly lifted off the floor. Keeping them flat on the floor puts stress on your back and doesn't give your upper body the best stretch, says certified personal trainer Karen Andes.

When you're in the plank pose, keep your back straight and don't let your hips sag or lift. Also, widen the space between your shoulder blades so they don't squeeze together, Andes says.

If you have any wrist problems such as carpal tunnel syndrome, arthritis, or osteoporosis, you should check with your doctor before trying this series of yoga poses.

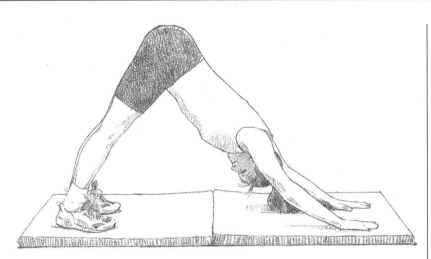

STEP 2: Tuck your toes under your feet so that your toes are on the floor and your heels are off the floor. Inhale and press your hips and buttocks upward as you straighten your legs. Exhale and gently push your heels down, keeping them slightly lifted off the floor. To help keep your legs straight, tense the muscles just above your knees. Bring your head downward so your ears are between your arms. Your arms should be completely straight, with the weight of your body evenly distributed between them. You should feel a good stretch throughout your whole torso. Hold this yoga pose, called the downward-facing dog, for 10 deep breaths.

Key things to remember
- Lift heels off floor slightly
- Keep legs straight
- Keep ears between arms
- Keep arms straight
- Contract muscles above knees

▶ **TAKE IT
TO THE MAX**
You can add a number of variations to the basic yoga poses of the modified pushup to make them more challenging, says certified personal trainer Karen Andes. First, you can bend your elbows in the downward-facing-dog pose to lower your head closer to the floor. Then straighten your arms when you move to the plank pose.

While in the plank position, lift your right leg off the floor so it's parallel to the floor, making sure to keep it straight. Then lower your right leg to the floor and lift your left leg.

Instead of returning to the starting position on all fours after the plank pose, first go back to the downward-facing dog for 10 more breaths, then return to the starting position.

(continued)

THE EXERCISES

Modified Pushup—Continued

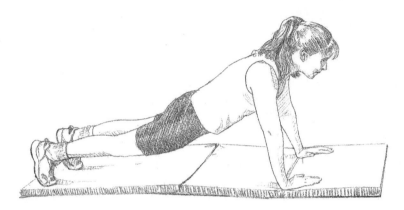

STEP 3: Without moving your hands or feet, and without bending your elbows, pivot your torso forward by lowering your buttocks and bringing your chest over your hands so that you're in the same position as you would be at the top of a pushup. If you find that you are not ending up with your hands in this exact position, it's okay to adjust them. Your body should form a diagonal line from your feet to your head. Make sure your hips don't sag, and keep your thighs and calves tensed and straight. Hold this yoga position, called the plank pose, for 10 deep breaths. Then return to the starting position on your hands and knees.

Key things to remember
• Don't let hips sag
• Align hands with shoulders
• Form diagonal line from feet to head
• Contract calves and thighs

THE STRETCHES

Doorway Stretch

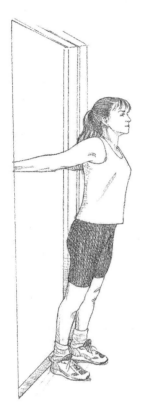

▶ WHAT IT DOES

Lengthens your chest and shoulder muscles

▶ HOW TO DO IT

Stand about a foot in front of an open door, with your feet hip-width apart. Hold on to both sides of the doorjamb, with your hands behind you and just below shoulder level. Gently lean forward with your chest so that your body, from your feet to your head, forms a diagonal line. Make sure not to lock your elbows or your knees, and don't let your heels lift off the floor. As you let your weight move forward, press your shoulders down so that they don't scrunch up around your ears. Hold the stretch for 30 seconds.

Key things to remember
- Keep hands just below shoulder level
- Form diagonal line from feet to head
- Don't lift heels
- Press shoulders down
- Don't lock elbows
- Don't lock knees

▶ DESKTOP TRAINER

Wall Pushup

Here's a simple way to give your chest muscles a workout at the office, says Lisa Womack, associate director of the Cardiac Health and Fitness Memorial Gym at the University of Virginia in Charlottesville. Stand facing a wall in your office area, about 2 feet away, with your feet hip-width apart. To start, extend your arms straight out from your body at chest height so that your palms are flat against the wall, shoulder-width apart. Do a standing pushup against the wall by bending your elbows so that your chest is close to the wall and your elbows are pointing downward. Then push yourself back to the starting position. Keep the rest of your body still and straight so that just your arms do the work.

REAL-LIFE SCENARIO

She'd Rather Lift Playing Cards

Eleanor, 50, has just had a call from her 28-year-old daughter, Samantha. Samantha has joined a brand-new health club, and she wants her mother to go with her. It's her chance to see more of her mom, and it's a great way for both of them to get healthier and into shape for the swimsuit season. But Eleanor is convinced that this health-club business isn't for her. She walks on the weekends, and that's enough. All those machines and heavy weights are fine for youngsters, but she can't see their point for a woman in middle age. What does she need a lot of muscles for, anyway? If she needs to lift something really heavy, she asks her husband to do it. She'd love to see more of her daughter, of course, but maybe they could join a bridge club together. Is Eleanor right? Or is she missing out on something?

Eleanor may want to reconsider her daughter's proposal. She may be missing a good bet. There's just as much of a reason to exercise at 50 as there is at 28. Eleanor surely knows that looking better, feeling stronger, being healthier, and raising self-esteem are not the exclusive concerns of the young.

In fact, there's at least one reason why strength training is even more worthwhile for Eleanor now than it was 20 years ago: Weight-bearing exercise strengthens bones, offsetting the increased risk of osteoporosis that comes after menopause. Eleanor is already helping her cause with her weekly walks. But they're not enough. If she walks more often—say, five times a week—and adds a couple days of simple weight workouts, she'll be doing her bones as well as her heart and muscles a big favor.

Still, she's right to recognize that there's a difference between what's "fine for youngsters" and what's right for her. She should realize that just because she'd be going to the health club with Samantha doesn't mean that she'd be exercising at the same pace or intensity as her daughter—or even doing the same things. That's why "all those machines" are adjustable. And not all of the weights are heavy. A good way for Eleanor to overcome her fear of the new health-club atmosphere is to take advantage of a credentialed professional, one who understands the middle-age body, to set her up with a routine that's just right for her.

Samantha can help her mom overcome the misconception that the health club isn't for her by introducing her to (or at least showing her pictures of) women her mom's age who have shaped up with weight training. But Samantha may have to accept that her mom may find more motivation in exercising with women her own age than in working out alongside of her daughter. She may even prefer to get some basic equipment and tone at home. Those are perfectly fine options and should be encouraged. As for seeing more of each other, well, Eleanor is right about that—there's always bridge club.

Expert Consulted
Carol Goldberg, Ph.D.
Clinical psychologist
President of Getting Ahead Programs, a corporation offering workshops on stress management,
*   health, and wellness*
New York City

Shoulders You Can Bare

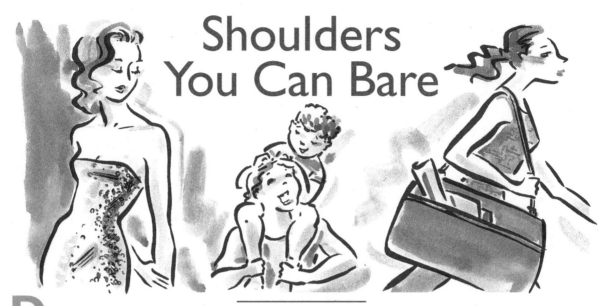

Do you know which legendary Hollywood diva was pumping iron to make her shoulders look great in a halter-top dress, long before it was fashionable to exercise?

Marilyn Monroe.

That's right. She wasn't born with those strong, shapely shoulders. She earned them. And so can you.

From lifting boxes or carrying a briefcase to hanging new curtains or putting luggage into an overhead compartment, we depend on our shoulders every day. We even find time to let friends cry on our shoulders. So what's the best way to keep those shoulders strong enough to handle these tasks by day *and* look great in a strapless dress by night?

First, you need to work the three deltoid muscles that form the front, middle, and back of each shoulder cap. Then, you also need to strengthen the deeper muscles that attach to the shoulder girdle and form the rotator cuff—they're what let you rotate your arm when you throw a softball, toss a Frisbee, or hit a tennis serve.

Your shoulders, especially your rotator cuffs, are vulnerable to overuse injuries caused by repetitive motion, explains Jennifer Layne, an exercise physiologist at Tufts University in Boston. Golfers, baseball pitchers, and tennis players are especially prone to rotator cuff injuries.

Arthritis and bursitis are common shoulder conditions that often affect athletes and older adults, Layne says. Arthritis is the gradual breakdown of cartilage in the joints, which leads to pain and stiffness. Bursitis occurs when the bursa, a sac of fluid that acts as a cushion between tendon and bone, becomes inflamed. If you have chronic shoulder pain, it may be either arthritis or bursitis. Make sure you get it checked out before starting a strength-training program, Layne cautions.

The exercises in this chapter work the three muscles in your shoulder cap as well as your rotator cuff, so you'll strengthen the muscles that you can see and those that you can't. If you tone your upper-back muscles along with your shoulders, before long you'll be snipping those foam shoulder pads out of your shirts and dresses. And here's a bonus: As your shoulders and back become toned, your upper body will look broader—making your waist appear slimmer.

THE EXERCISES

Seated Fly

▶ WHAT IT DOES

Strengthens the middle of
your shoulder

▶ IT'S GOOD FOR:

 bowling

 softball

 swimming

 volleyball

▶ GO FOR YOUR GOAL

Drop a Dress Size: *Two
sets of 10 reps, without
dumbbells, for 1 to 2
weeks; then two sets of 10
reps with 1- to 2-pound
dumbbells*

Shape Up: *Three sets of
8 reps with 2- to 5-pound
dumbbells*

Maintain: *Two to three
sets of 8 to 12 reps with 5-
to 8-pound dumbbells*

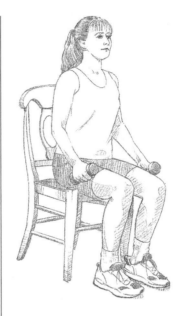

STEP 1: Sit in an armless chair, with
good posture so that you're not
slouching and your abdominal and back
muscles are supporting your trunk.
Place your feet flat on the floor, about
hip-width apart. Keeping your arms
against your body, hold one dumbbell in
each hand, with your palms facing your
thighs and your elbows slightly bent. If
possible, check your position in a
mirror.

Key things to remember

• Bend elbows
• Maintain good posture
• Keep palms facing thighs
• Keep arms against body

LISTEN TO YOUR BODY

When doing a seated fly, make sure you lift from
your shoulders. That's where you want to feel the effort. "Your forearms are really just along for the ride,"
says exercise physiologist Jennifer Layne. But don't let your forearms or the dumbbells lag behind. As you lift, keep your entire
arm—from your upper arm to your hand—in the same plane,
with your the whole arm reaching shoulder height at the end of
the lift.

It's important to maintain the same bend in your elbow from

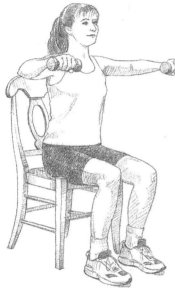

STEP 2: Before lifting the dumbbells, bring your shoulder blades together slightly. While exhaling, take two counts to lift both arms until they're out to your sides at shoulder height, making sure to keep your elbows bent. At the end of the lift, your arms, your elbows, and the dumbbells should all be at shoulder height and parallel to the floor. Hold this position for one count. Then inhale as you take four counts to lower the dumbbells back to the starting position. Repeat.

Key things to remember
- Keep elbows slightly bent
- Lift arms and dumbbells to shoulder height, parallel to floor
- Keep wrists straight
- Don't hunch shoulders

▶ **TAKE IT TO THE MAX**

To make the seated fly a bit more difficult, open the angles of your bent arms so that they're closer to being straight. Just make sure they're not completely straight; you still need slight bends. Make the adjustment while in the starting position, and maintain it throughout the exercise.

start to finish. That bend is for protection: Having your arms straight out at your sides puts a lot of pressure on your shoulder joints, Layne says. You want your arms to be bent at about 110-degree angles, that is, slightly more open than right angles. Also, be sure not to hunch up your shoulders as you lift your arms.

When choosing your weights for this exercise, think light. "You should start lower than you think you can handle," Layne says. To make sure they have it down, she suggests, beginners may even want to practice the move without dumbbells before adding weights.

THE EXERCISES

Seated Overhead Press

▶ **WHAT IT DOES**
Works the fronts and backs of your shoulders as well as your upper back

▶ **IT'S GOOD FOR:**
All sports

▶ **GO FOR YOUR GOAL**

Drop a Dress Size: *Two sets of 10 reps with 1- to 3-pound dumbbells*

Shape Up: *Three sets of 8 reps with 3- to 5-pound dumbbells*

Maintain: *Two to three sets of 8 to 12 reps with 5- to 10-pound dumbbells*

STEP 1: Sit upright toward the front of a chair, with your feet flat on the floor and about hip-width apart. Raise your forearms so that your hands are even with your shoulders. Keep your upper arms snug against the sides of your body, with your elbows pointing down. Your forearms should be just to the outside of your body. Hold one dumbbell in each hand, with your palms facing away from you. One head of each dumbbell should be just in front of each shoulder. Keep your wrists in a straight line with the backs of your hands so that you don't let your wrists bend. This is the starting position.

Key things to remember
• Keep lower back straight and supported
• Keep upper arms against body
• Point elbows down
• Keep wrists straight
• Keep palms facing away from you

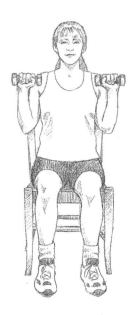

 LISTEN TO YOUR BODY

A common mistake with the seated overhead press is to let your wrists bend back as you lift, says exercise physiologist Jennifer Layne. Be sure that your wrists and the backs of your hands are straight and in line with one another. "It's a good idea to recheck your hand position after each rep so that your hands do not drift backward," she says.

You also need to make sure you're not leaning or arching your torso backward to get the weights up higher. As you lift the dumbbells, remember to keep them in the same vertical plane in front of your shoulders as they were in the starting position. Don't lift them

STEP 2: Exhale as you press the dumbbells straight up for two counts. Fully extend your arms, but don't lock your elbows. Keep your wrists and your arms straight and in line with each other. Hold for one count at the top of the position. Then inhale and take four counts to lower the dumbbells back to the starting position. Repeat.

Key things to remember
- Don't lock elbows
- Don't bend wrists
- Hold dumbbells slightly in front of body, not directly overhead

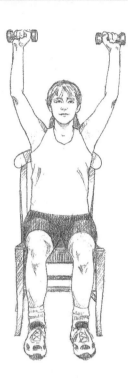

▶ **TAKE IT TO THE MAX**

You can give the middles of your shoulders and your upper back more of a workout by changing the seated overhead press slightly. Start in the same position, with the dumbbells just in front of your shoulders. When you lift the weights, bring them directly over your head instead of lifting them so they're slightly in front of your body. Just make sure that the weights never go *behind* your head. At the top of the move, bring the dumbbells together so that the inside heads of the weights touch each other. When you lower the weights, bring them back to the original starting position.

Because this variation is more challenging and not as shoulder-friendly, says exercise physiologist Jennifer Layne, if you have any shoulder problems such as arthritis, tendonitis, or a past injury to a rotator cuff, stick with the basic version of the exercise.

directly up over your head; keep them slightly in front of your body so they're in line with your nose, Layne says.

To keep an eye on your form, it's a good idea to watch yourself in a mirror when you do this exercise. "As the reps progress in the set, there's a tendency for your elbows to drift away from your body and for your hands to move in toward your chest," Layne says. When you return to the starting position, make sure your upper arms are against your sides, with your elbows pointing straight down. One head of each dumbbell should be just in front of each shoulder, with the other ball to the outside of that shoulder.

THE EXERCISES

Upright Row

▶ WHAT IT DOES

Tones the fronts and middles of your shoulders as well as your biceps and forearms

▶ IT'S GOOD FOR:

 bowling

 golf

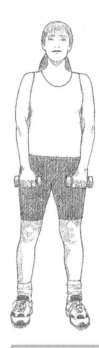 tennis

▶ GO FOR YOUR GOAL

Drop a Dress Size: *Two sets of 10 reps with 1- to 5-pound dumbbells*

Shape Up: *Three sets of 8 reps with 5- to 8-pound dumbbells*

Maintain: *Two to three sets of 8 to 12 reps with 8- to 12-pound dumbbells*

STEP 1: Stand with good posture and with your feet hip-width apart. Hold one dumbbell in each hand, and extend your arms straight down in front of you, with your palms facing your body and the dumbbells resting against the centers of your thighs. This is the starting position. Do this exercise in front of a mirror if you can.

Key things to remember

- Don't lock knees
- Don't shrug shoulders
- Don't lock elbows
- Hold dumbbells against centers of thighs
- Keep palms facing body

LISTEN TO YOUR BODY

The most important piece of equipment for the upright-row exercise is a mirror. "I don't know why, but many beginning weight lifters lose all sense of body awareness when they do this exercise," says exercise physiologist Jennifer Layne. "Watching yourself in the mirror really is the key to achieving proper technique."

To get the most out of this exercise, you should watch out for a number of common mistakes. First, be sure that you're not shrugging your shoulders up to your ears to lift the weights. Instead, keep your elbows out to the sides and lift your elbows up so that your hands follow, Layne says. Bringing your shoulder blades together slightly before you lift the dumbbells will also help.

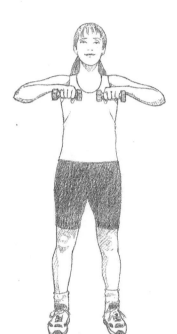

STEP 2: Bring your shoulder blades together slightly before lifting the dumbbells. Then exhale and take two counts to lift the dumbbells straight up, keeping them close to your body while you lift. Focus on lifting from the backs of your shoulders and leading with your elbows. At the end of the lift, your upper arms should be at shoulder-height and parallel to the floor, elbows pointing out to the sides. Your forearms will be slightly lower than your upper arms, with the dumbbells in front of your chest. Hold this position for one count. Then inhale as you take four counts to lower the dumbbells back to the starting position. Repeat.

Key things to remember
- Press shoulders down
- Keep upper arms parallel to floor
- Hold dumbbells in front of chest
- Don't curl wrists

Another thing to watch out for is that your upper arms should not go above shoulder height and that the dumbbells should come up only to your chest—no higher, Layne says. As you lift the weights, make sure to keep them close to your body. "They should be so close that they almost graze your body."

You should also check that you're lifting the dumbbells straight up, as if they're on rails or tracks. Don't worry about keeping the dumbbells parallel to the floor, Layne says. The more important thing is that your wrists and hands stay in the same position throughout the move. You shouldn't roll your hands back or curl your wrists. "It may help to pretend that you're lifting a bar, rather than two hand weights," she suggests.

THE EXERCISES

External Shoulder Rotation

▶ **WHAT IT DOES**
Strengthens your rotator cuff

▶ **IT'S GOOD FOR:**

 bowling

 cycling

 golf

 tennis

▶ **GO FOR YOUR GOAL**

Drop a Dress Size: *Two sets of 10 reps on each side empty-handed or with a 1-pound dumbbell*

Shape Up: *Three sets of 8 reps on each side with a 1- to 3-pound dumbbell*

Maintain: *Two to three sets of 8 to 12 reps on each side with a 3- to 5-pound dumbbell*

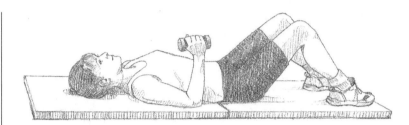

STEP 1: Lie face-up on a mat, with your knees bent and the small of your back against the floor. Your feet should be flat on the floor, about hip-width apart. Keep the upper part of your right arm snug against your body. Bend your elbow so that your forearm is perpendicular to the floor and forms a 90-degree angle with your upper arm. Hold a dumbbell in your right hand with your palm facing your body and your knuckles facing up. If you do this move without a dumbbell, make a fist so that your knuckles face up. This is the starting position.

Key things to remember
• Press lower back against floor
• Hold upper arm against body
• Bend forearm perpendicular to floor
• Keep palm facing body; keep knuckles face-up

 LISTEN TO YOUR BODY

One key to doing the external shoulder rotation correctly is to keep your lower back and shoulder blades pressed to the floor as you lower the dumbbell, says exercise physiologist Jennifer Layne. When you lower the weight, don't force your arm closer to the floor than it's able to go—and don't bend your wrist to bring the dumbbell closer to the floor.

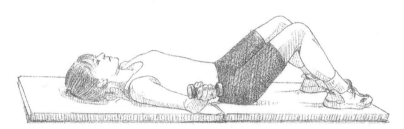

STEP 2: Keeping your upper arm against your body and your wrist straight, exhale and, for two counts, move your forearm straight out to the side as if you were trying to touch the floor with the back of your hand. Go as far as you can without cocking your wrist. You may be able to go only a few inches. Hold the position for one count, then inhale as you take four counts to raise the dumbbell to the starting position. Once you've completed a set with your right arm, switch and do a set with your left. Repeat.

Key things to remember
- Keep wrist straight
- Hold upper arm against body
- Lower forearm toward floor as far as is comfortable

If you feel strain or discomfort in your upper arm, that means you're coming down too far. For your next rep, bring your arm down only as far as you can without feeling that discomfort. If you're lowering the weight only a few inches toward the floor, you're still benefiting from the exercise, Layne says. After a few sessions, you'll probably be able to move it farther. "For some people, going halfway to the floor is going to be a real achievement."

THE EXERCISES

Port de Bras

▶ **WHAT IT DOES**
Targets the middles of
your shoulders

▶ **GO FOR YOUR GOAL**
Drop a Dress Size: *8 to
10 reps*
Shape Up: *10 to 12 reps*
Maintain: *12 to 16 reps*

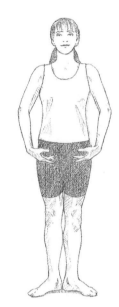

STEP 1: Start in ballet first position, with your toes turned to 2 and 10 o'clock and with proper posture, as shown. Your thighs, calves, and heels should touch, and your abs and buttocks should be tight. Press your shoulders down; and hold your hands in front of your thighs, with your elbows slightly rounded. Hold this position for two counts; then move into the next position.

Key things to remember
• Stand with heels together
• Tighten abs
• Squeeze buttocks
• Press shoulders down
• Keep arms rounded

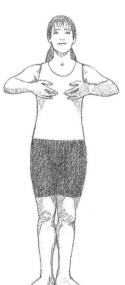

STEP 2: Keep your arms rounded and your shoulders down. Raise your arms, leading with your elbows. At the end of the move, your palms should be in front of your chest, just below shoulder height. Hold for two counts, then move right into the next position.

Key things to remember
• Hold palms in front of chest
• Press shoulders down
• Keep arms rounded

STEP 3: Bring your arms out to the sides so that there are slight bends in your elbows and your arms remain just below shoulder height. As you open your arms, your shoulder blades will come together slightly. Take three counts to complete this last position.

Key things to remember
• Hold arms just below shoulder height
• Keep elbows slightly bent
• Press shoulder blades together

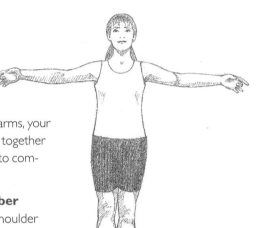

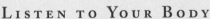

▶ TAKE IT TO THE MAX
To make the port de bras even more intense, you can strap ankle weights onto your wrists, says certified personal trainer Karen Andes. She suggests using 1- to 2-pound weights if your goal is to drop a dress size, 2- to 4-pound weights to shape up, and 4- to 5-pound weights to maintain your fitness level.

LISTEN TO YOUR BODY

If your neck feels tense or it doesn't feel like your shoulders are working very hard when you do the port de bras, make sure you're not shrugging your shoulders, says certified personal trainer Karen Andes. "To get the most out of this exercise, pull your shoulders down and back slightly, as if you have two ankle weights draped over your shoulders, holding them down," she says.

To help you achieve the graceful arms of a dancer, think of each arm as extending from your shoulder to the tips of your fingers. Relax your fingers so they look elegant, as if you were holding a sherry glass between your thumb and middle finger, Andes suggests. Don't tense them up into a claw.

Even though this dance move focuses on the shoulders, you still need to maintain good posture and contract your abdominal muscles to support your trunk, Andes adds.

THE STRETCHES

Overhead Stretch

▶ **DESKTOP TRAINER**

Tension Reliever

Many women with desk jobs tend to sit with their shoulders hunched up and rounded forward, which can make for a real pain in the neck. This shoulder position causes tightness in the neck and upper-back muscles that attach to the shoulders. Here's a quick stretch from exercise physiologist Jennifer Layne to help relieve that built-up muscle tension.

Sit in your chair with good posture and your feet flat on the floor. Keeping your shoulders down and back, bend your neck and move your right ear toward your right shoulder. You should feel a good stretch on the left side of your neck and upper back. Hold the stretch for 30 seconds, then move your left ear to your left shoulder to stretch your right side.

▶ **WHAT IT DOES**

Stretches your shoulder muscles, rotator cuffs, and upper arms

▶ **HOW TO DO IT**

Sit on a chair with your back straight and your feet flat on the floor, about hip-width apart. Raise your arms straight up so they're slightly in front of your body, not directly over your head. Interlace your fingers and press your shoulder blades together slightly. Then push upward until you feel a comfortable stretch in your shoulders and upper arms, making sure not to shrug your shoulders. If you're very flexible, you can move your arms so they're directly over your head, but do not bring your arms behind your head. Hold the stretch for 30 seconds.

Key things to remember
• Don't lock elbows
• Press shoulders down
• Maintain good posture
• Interlace fingers
• Hold arms slightly in front of body

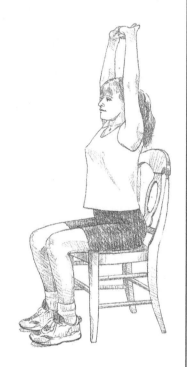

Arms That Will Knock Them Out

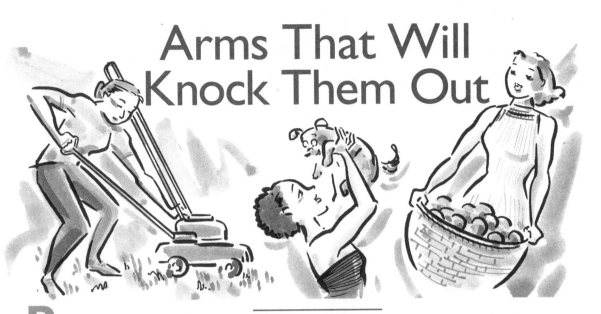

Remember when your best friend got married? The girl with whom you went through grade school, swapped first-kiss stories, and skipped rope? Your happiness for her knew no bounds.

Then she asked you to be in her wedding party. The first thing out of your mouth after "Yes" was almost certainly "What kind of dresses do you have in mind?"

Of course, what you were really thinking was "Please don't make me wear a frilly chartreuse dress that doesn't have any sleeves!"

It's sad but true. The love we have for our friends only goes so far, and it can stop at the altar, especially when it means exposing some upper-arm flab.

That flab is easy to come by. Beside using our arms to push ourselves out of a chair or reaching up to stack things on a high shelf, Layne says, we don't often use our triceps in a way that will strengthen and tone them.

Getting rid of those jiggly upper arms takes a one-two punch. "This is an area where fat tends to accumulate," says Jennifer Layne, an exercise physiologist at Tufts University in Boston. So the first punch is to lose some extra pounds through diet and exercise. Once you shed that layer of arm fat, you'll be able to see the underlying muscles. The knockout punch, says Layne, is to give those muscles more shape and definition through toning exercises.

There are three sets of muscles that you'll need to work on. The first is the biceps, which are the muscles in the fronts of your upper arms. These muscles bend your elbow joints. The second is the triceps—the muscles in the backs of your upper arms that straighten out your arms. "Women tend to have weak triceps because we don't use these muscles a lot in our day-to-day lives," Layne explains. Finally, there's a few smaller muscles called elbow flexors, which stretch from your upper arms to your forearms. They help bend and rotate your elbows.

The workout that we've put together targets all of these muscles, so you'll soon be carrying heavier loads with ease. Your bowling and tennis games will improve. And best of all, you won't want to keep your upper arms under wraps.

THE EXERCISES

Arm Curl

▶ **WHAT IT DOES**
Works your biceps and elbow flexors

▶ **IT'S GOOD FOR:**
All sports

▶ **GO FOR YOUR GOAL**

Drop a Dress Size: *Two sets of 10 reps on each side with 1- to 5-pound dumbbells*

Shape Up: *Three sets of 8 reps on each side with 5- to 10-pound dumbbells*

Maintain: *Two to three sets of 8 to 12 reps on each side with 10- to 15-pound dumbbells*

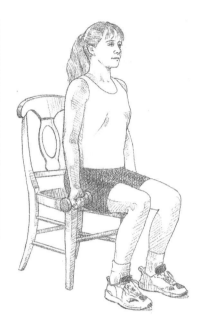

STEP 1: Sit on the edge of a chair with good posture so that you're not slouching and your abdominal and back muscles are supporting your trunk. Your feet should be flat on the floor, about hip-width apart. Hold a dumbbell in each hand so that your elbows and upper arms are snug against the sides of your body. Your forearms should be extended straight down at your sides, with your palms facing forward. This is the starting position.

Key things to remember
• Maintain good posture
• Hold upper arms and elbows against body
• Hold palms facing forward
• Don't lock elbows

LISTEN TO YOUR BODY

One key to the arm-curl exercise is to make sure you don't move your elbow forward as you lift the dumbbell. Keep your upper arm and elbow still and pressed against your side throughout the move so that your elbow points down, not forward. "It may help to pretend that you have a winning lottery ticket between your arm and side, and don't want to let it fall," says exercise physiologist Jennifer Layne.

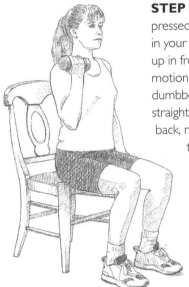

STEP 2: Keeping your elbows gently pressed against your sides, raise the dumbbell in your right hand by bringing your forearm up in front of your shoulder in one smooth motion. Remember to exhale as you lift the dumbbell for two counts. Keep your wrist straight and your shoulders slightly down and back, not hunched up. At the end of the lift, the dumbbell should be in front of your shoulder, with your palm facing your shoulder. Hold for one count, then take four counts to slowly lower the dumbbell to the starting position. Repeat with your left arm, and continue alternating arms with each repetition until you've completed your sets.

Key things to remember

- Keep elbows against body
- Press shoulders down and back
- Don't curl wrist
- Raise dumbbell in front of shoulder
- Keep palm facing shoulder

A few more things to keep in mind: Your wrist should be straight and in line with the back of your hand, not curled, Layne says. If you find yourself ending the lift with the dumbbell in front of your chest instead of your shoulder (where it should be), you're probably crossing your arm over your body as you lift. To fix your form, make sure to lift the dumbbell straight up. Finally, don't lean back to help you lift the dumbbell—lift with your arm, and keep your torso straight and supported with your back and abdominal muscles, Layne says.

▶ **TAKE IT TO THE MAX**

Change the starting position of the arm curl, and you'll give the muscles in your forearms more of a workout. Instead of starting with your palms facing forward as shown, turn your arms in slightly so that your palms face your legs, says exercise physiologist Jennifer Layne. As in the basic arm curl, your arms should be straight down at your sides, but your elbows should not be locked.

Slowly raise your right dumbbell, gradually rotating your forearm as you lift, so that at the top of the lift your arm is in the same position as shown in the illustration—with the dumbbell in front of your shoulder and your palm facing your shoulder. Hold for one count. Slowly rotate your forearm as you lower the dumbbell, so that you return to the starting position with your palm facing your leg. Repeat with your left arm, and so on.

Triceps Kickback

▶ **WHAT IT DOES**
Tones your triceps

▶ **IT'S GOOD FOR:**

 bowling

SB softball

▶ **GO FOR YOUR GOAL**

Drop a Dress Size: *Two sets of 10 reps on each side with a 1- to 5-pound dumbbell*

Shape Up: *Three sets of 8 reps on each side with a 5- to 8-pound dumbbell*

Maintain: *Two to three sets of 8 to 12 reps on each side with a 8- to 12-pound dumbbell*

STEP 1: Lean over a chair with your right hand on the seat for support. Your arm should be straight, but your elbow should not be locked. Place your right knee and shin on the seat. Keep your back flat and look straight down at the floor so that your neck is in line with your spine. Hold the dumbbell in your left hand, with your palm facing your body and your wrist straight. Keep your left arm, your elbow, and the upper part of your left arm close to your body. Bend your elbow so that your forearm forms a right angle with your upper arm. Your left leg should be straight, with your toes facing front, but your knee should not be locked. This is your starting position.

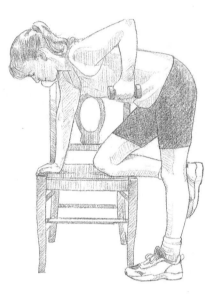

Key things to remember
• Don't lock elbow
• Keep shoulder and wrist in line
• Keep back straight
• Keep neck and spine in line
• Don't lock knee
• Hold upper arm and elbow against body

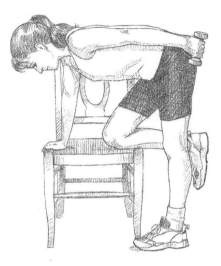

STEP 2: Exhale for two counts as you straighten your left arm by moving your forearm backward and upward so that it's even with your shoulder. At the end of the lift, your arm should be straight, but your elbow should not be locked. Be careful not to lift your forearm higher than your shoulder, and make sure to keep your elbow and upper arm pressed against your body as you lift the dumbbell. At the end of the lift, hold the position for one count. Then inhale as you take four counts to lower the dumbbell back to the starting position. After completing a set, repeat the exercise with your right arm.

Key things to remember
- Keep upper arm and elbow against body
- Lift forearm to shoulder height
- Keep palm facing body
- Don't lock elbow

LISTEN TO YOUR BODY

If your upper arm moves away from your body—or moves at all—when you lift the dumbbell, you won't get the full benefit from the triceps kickback, says exercise physiologist Jennifer Layne. "Only your forearm should move; your upper arm stays still."

Your elbow acts as the pivot for the movement, but otherwise does not move. "Some women let their elbows come up as they lift, which you don't want to do," Layne says.

You also don't want to rotate your forearm as you lift the dumbbell. A good way to check your form is to make sure your palm faces toward your body at the end of the lift. If it faces away from your body, you're rotating your forearm. To fix your form, concentrate on keeping your upper arm in the same position from start to finish.

Overhead Triceps Extension

▶ **WHAT IT DOES**
Strengthens your triceps

▶ **IT'S GOOD FOR:**

 swimming

tennis

▶ **GO FOR YOUR GOAL**

Drop a Dress Size: *Two sets of 10 reps with a 1- to 3-pound dumbbell*

Shape Up: *Three sets of 8 reps with a 3- to 5-pound dumbbell*

Maintain: *Two to three sets of 8 to 12 reps with a 5- to 10-pound dumbbell*

STEP 1: Begin by sitting in a chair with good posture and with your feet flat on the floor, about hip-width apart. Hold a dumbbell in your left hand. To get into the starting position, extend your left arm down at your side, with your palm facing in toward your thigh. Then lift the dumbbell straight over your head so that your left arm is fully extended and your palm faces in. Bend your elbow to lower the dumbbell behind the nape of your neck. This is the starting position for the exercise. Your wrist should be straight and in line with the back of your hand, and your elbow should point up as high as possible. Bring your right arm across your body to help support the upper part of your left arm. Keep your right arm and elbow close to your body, with your elbow pointing downward.

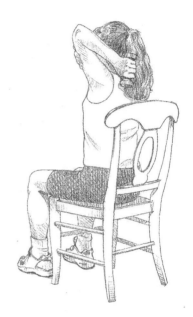

Key things to remember
- Keep wrist straight
- Point elbow up
- Support arm with other hand
- Keep back straight and supported
- Keep supporting arm close to body

STEP 2: Without moving your left elbow or upper arm, lift the dumbbell straight up so that your arm is fully extended. The palm of your hand should face in. Exhale for two counts as you lift the dumbbell, making sure not to lock your elbow at the end of the lift. Hold the fully extended position for one count. Then inhale as you take four counts to slowly lower the dumbbell back to the starting position.

Key things to remember
- Fully extend forearm
- Raise dumbbell over head
- Keep upper arm and elbow still
- Keep palm facing in
- Don't lock elbow

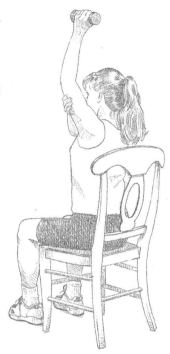

LISTEN TO YOUR BODY

While the overhead triceps extension is not as shoulder-friendly as some other exercises, it is very effective at toning the back of the arm, says exercise physiologist Jennifer Layne. But be aware: "It's wise to do the triceps kickback instead of this exercise if you feel pain or discomfort in your shoulder," Layne advises. This exercise can be challenging or inappropriate for women with shoulder limitations such as bursitis, arthritis, or rotator cuff injuries, she adds.

Even if you don't feel discomfort, this exercise may initially feel awkward. That's normal, assures Layne. You may not be flexible enough to point your elbow straight up in the starting position. In that case, your elbow may point out to the side a bit and may not be as high up as shown in the illustration, Layne says. As you become more flexible, you should be able to bring your elbow higher.

Two common mistakes are to lock your elbow at the end of the lift and to rotate your wrist or forearm as you lift the dumbbell. If you feel discomfort in your elbow, you're probably locking the joint, Layne says. To fix your form, don't straighten your arm as much. At the top of the move, leave a slight bend in your arm. When you lift and lower the dumbbell, be sure to bring your forearm and wrist straight up and down so that you're not rotating them, she adds.

THE EXERCISES

Modified Teapot Pose

▶ **WHAT IT DOES**
Shapes your triceps

▶ **GO FOR YOUR GOAL**

Drop a Dress Size: *6 to 8 reps on each side*

Shape Up: *8 to 10 reps on each side*

Maintain: *10 to 12 reps on each side*

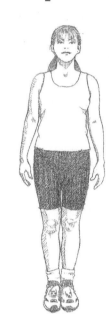

STEP 1: Start by standing up straight, with your feet together and your arms down at your sides. Look straight ahead and maintain good posture, with your shoulders pressed down.

Key things to remember
• Stand with feet together
• Hold arms down at sides
• Press shoulders down
• Look ahead

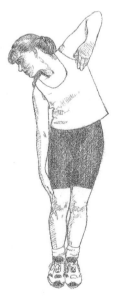

STEP 2: Keeping your weight centered over your feet, bend from your waist and extend your right arm downward so that your hand is against your leg and you're looking down over your right shoulder. Raise your left elbow upward, touching your fingertips to your outer chest. Keep your abdominal muscles tight to help support your lower back.

Key things to remember
• Reach down with fingers
• Point opposite elbow up
• Look down over shoulder
• Tighten abs
• Center weight over feet

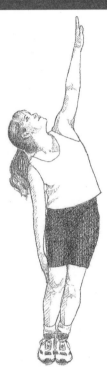

STEP 3: Extend your left arm straight up, with your palm facing away from you. Gently follow the movement of your arm with your head so that at the end of the move you're looking up at the tips of your fingers. Focus on reaching upward as high as you can with your fingers. Return to the starting position, and repeat the move by bending to your left. Continue alternating sides for each rep until you've completed all of the reps for your goal.

Key things to remember
- Hold palm facing away
- Look at fingertips
- Reach as high as you can

▶ **TAKE IT TO THE MAX**
To give your triceps a tougher workout, do the modified teapot pose with ankle weights strapped onto your wrists. Try using a 1- to 5-pound weight on each wrist, suggests certified personal trainer Karen Andes. Start with lighter weights, and gradually increase to heavier ones, she advises.

LISTEN TO YOUR BODY

If you feel discomfort in your hip or lower back when you do the modified teapot pose, you're probably leaning into your hip too far, says certified personal trainer Karen Andes. Try to keep your lower body as straight and still as possible. It may help to imagine that your arms stretch along a vertical axis running through the middle of your body, Andes says. Keeping your weight centered over your feet and tightening your abs should also help stabilize your back and lower body. As with many of the dance exercises, this uses a continuous, flowing movement, so the positions should all flow together.

Scratch-Your-Back Stretch

▶ **DESKTOP TRAINER**

Mock Arm Curl

This office exercise can give your biceps and elbow flexors a mini-workout. Sit close to your desk with your hands under it, palms facing up, says exercise physiologist Jennifer Layne. Push up on the desk with your hands, making sure to keep your elbows and upper arms against your sides. Be careful not to shrug your shoulders or hold your breath. You should feel your biceps and forearms contracting. Hold for 10 to 30 seconds. Relax, then repeat for three sets of eight reps.

▶ **WHAT IT DOES**

Increases flexibility of your triceps

▶ **HOW TO DO IT**

The position for this stretch is the same as the starting position for the overhead triceps extension, but you don't use a dumbbell. Sit in a chair with good posture and with your feet flat on the floor, about hip-width apart. Point your left elbow toward the ceiling, with your forearm down behind you so that your palm is just behind the base of your neck and your fingers point downward. Hold the back of your left upper arm with your right hand by bringing your right arm across your body. You can increase the stretch by trying to reach farther down your back with your fingers. You can also put gentle pressure on your left upper arm with your right hand to help you reach farther. Hold the stretch for 30 seconds, then repeat with your right arm.

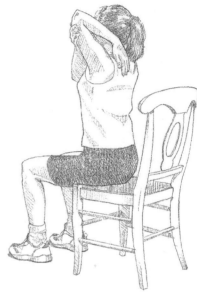

Key things to remember

- Point elbow up
- Press arm gently to increase stretch
- Keep arm and elbow close to body
- Reach down back with fingers

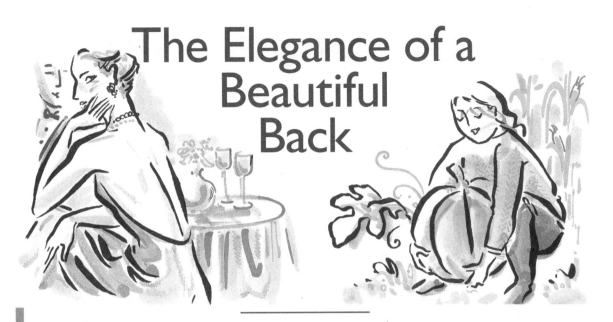

The Elegance of a Beautiful Back

It takes more than a pretty smile and a beautiful gown to be truly elegant. Just ask Miss Spain. During the 1999 Miss Universe pageant, the emcee asked her this question: "As a clothing designer, which do you think is more important, the front of a dress or the back?"

"The front," she answered, "because you should look a person in the eyes." Then, on the emcee's cue, she turned around to reveal her backless gown, drawing a roar of cheers and applause from the crowd.

She was named second runner-up.

A woman's back can be very alluring, but it's also vulnerable to injury. Eighty percent of adults experience back pain at some point in their lives, says Jennifer Layne, an exercise physiologist at Tufts University in Boston. "The stronger your back is, the less likely you are to injure it," she says.

Toned back muscles also make lifting and carrying heavy items easier and safer; and they are critical for proper posture, which helps support your internal organs, Layne says. In terms of bone health—a particular concern for women—strengthening your back helps prevent osteoporosis by maintaining the bone in your spine.

For a strong, beautiful back, you need to work the muscles in your upper, middle, and lower back, namely the trapezius, rhomboid, and latissimus dorsi. You also need to strengthen the three muscles that run along your spine, called the erector spinae. They help support and control the movement of your vertebrae. The exercises in this chapter target all of these muscle groups for a complete back workout.

To further protect against back injuries, here are some tips from Layne. When you lift something—whether it's a bag of groceries or a dumbbell—make sure you keep the object close to your body. Bend your knees when lifting, so you use your legs, hips, and buttocks as well as your back. If you spend long periods sitting or driving, make sure your seat is comfortable and supports your lower back. Avoid wearing heels that are more than 2 inches high; they can cause your lower back to arch. And when you do weight-bearing exercises, always check your body alignment to make sure your back is not arched.

THE EXERCISES

Land Swim

▶ **WHAT IT DOES**

Works your entire back, especially the muscles that run up and down your spine

▶ **IT'S GOOD FOR:**

 cycling

 dancing

 golf

 swimming

▶ **GO FOR YOUR GOAL**

Drop a Dress Size: *Two sets of 10 reps on each side*

Shape Up: *Three sets of 8 reps on each side*

Maintain: *Two to three sets of 8 to 12 reps on each side*

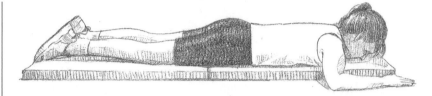

STEP 1: Lie face-down on a mat with your legs straight and your toes pointed so that the laces of your sneakers face the floor. Bend your right arm at a 90-degree angle as if you were making half of a goal post, and extend your left arm down at your side. Your right palm should face down, while your left palm faces up.

Key things to remember
- Place palm down
- Place palm up
- Face shoelaces down
- Bend arm at 90-degree angle

LISTEN TO YOUR BODY

One thing that you need to look out for with the land swim is that your neck and spine should always align, says exercise physiologist Jennifer Layne. To avoid rocking your head backward and out of alignment, keep your nose down so that it's always facing the floor, she suggests.

Even though it's called the land swim, you don't swim or kick when you do this exercise. The move is very slow and controlled so that you don't strain your back. You also want to make sure that you bring your leg straight up. "Keep the front of your hips pressed flat against the floor to effectively target your lower back," suggests Layne.

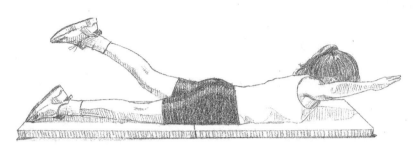

STEP 2: Exhale as you raise your left leg and bent right arm as high as you comfortably can. Your leg should be straight, with your toes pointed, so that you're lifting your entire leg from your hip to your toes. If you're strong enough, you can also raise your shoulders and upper chest off the floor to get more of a workout. Take two counts to raise your arm, chest, and leg, hold the position for one count, then lower for two counts to return to the starting position. Complete one set, then raise your left arm, your chest, and your right leg.

Key things to remember
- Don't tilt head back
- Keep hips pressed flat against floor
- Point toes
- Face shoelaces down

▶ **TAKE IT TO THE MAX**
You can make the land swim a bit more challenging by extending your working arm straight out in front of you, instead of bending it at a 90-degree angle. The palm of your working arm should be flat on the floor, with your upper arm by your ear. Place your other arm straight down at your side, palm up. Do the exercise as shown: Lift your arm, shoulders, and upper chest as well as your opposite leg. Keep the arm that you're lifting straight and fully extended as you raise it off the floor.

You should feel the effort in your upper and lower back, but you should not feel pain, Layne says. "Women are sometimes alarmed or concerned to feel something in their lower back, but it's a muscle like any other. If they don't feel like they're being challenged, then the muscle isn't getting worked."

Women are also surprised that such a small movement—for some, it's only a few inches—can be so difficult. "Some women find that this is the most intense exercise in their program because their backs are so weak," Layne says. If you keep working at it, this exercise will become easier. As your back gets stronger, you should be able to lift your leg and upper chest higher off the floor.

THE EXERCISES

Dumbbell Row

▶ **WHAT IT DOES**
Strengthens your upper
back and the back of your
shoulder

▶ **IT'S GOOD FOR:**

 bowling

 golf

 tennis

▶ **GO FOR YOUR GOAL**

Drop a Dress Size: *Two
sets of 10 reps on each side
with a 1- to 5-pound dumbbell*

Shape Up: *Three sets of
8 reps on each side with a
5- to 10-pound dumbbell*

Maintain: *Two to three
sets of 8 to 12 reps on
each side with a 10- to 12-
pound dumbbell*

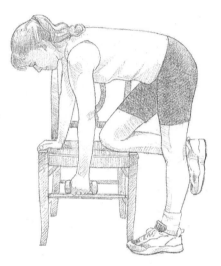

STEP 1: Lean over a chair
with your right arm on the seat
for support. Your arm should
be straight, but your elbow
should not be locked. Place
your right knee and shin on
the seat. Keep your back flat
and look straight down at the
floor so that your neck is in
line with your spine. Hold the
dumbbell in your left hand,
with your palm facing your
body and your wrist straight.
Keep your left arm fully extended, with your hand in line
with your shoulder and your elbow slightly bent. Your left leg should be
straight, with your toes facing front, but your knee should not be locked.
This is the starting position.

Key things to remember
• Don't lock elbows
• Look down
• Don't lock knee
• Keep neck in line with spine
• Keep back flat

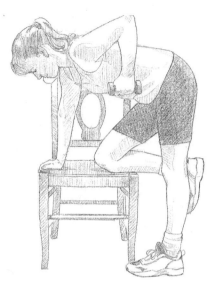

STEP 2: Before lifting the dumbbell, inhale and bring your shoulder blades together slightly so that your back will stay flat as you lift. Then exhale as you lift the dumbbell straight up for two counts. Keep your left arm, your elbow, and the dumbbell close to your body as you lift. Hold the dumbbell at the top of the move for one count, then inhale as you take four counts to lower the dumbbell back to the starting position. After you've completed a set with your left arm, repeat the exercise with your right arm.

Key things to remember
- Keep dumbbell close to body
- Keep back flat
- Bring elbow up past body

LISTEN TO YOUR BODY

Make sure you're in proper position for the dumbbell row. "It is important to fully extend your torso so that your back is flat, not rounded," says exercise physiologist Jennifer Layne. If you're tall, you may need to use a weight bench or a piano bench instead of a chair, so you can elongate your back.

A common mistake is using a dumbbell that's too light so that you pull up as if you're starting a lawn mower. "You need to make sure that you're challenging yourself with the weight for this exercise," Layne says.

When you lift the dumbbell, keep your arm, your elbow, and the weight snug against your body. That will help you get the most out of the exercise and will prevent upper-back or neck strain, Layne says. When you lower the dumbbell, make sure you don't lock your elbow as you fully extend your arm. Doing so puts a lot of stress on your elbow and shoulder joints, she explains.

THE EXERCISES

Pullover

▶ **WHAT IT DOES**

Targets your upper back as well as your chest muscles

▶ **IT'S GOOD FOR:**

 softball

 swimming

tennis

▶ **GO FOR YOUR GOAL**

Drop a Dress Size: *Two sets of 10 reps with a 3- to 5-pound dumbbell*

Shape Up: *Three sets of 8 reps with a 5- to 8-pound dumbbell*

Maintain: *Two to three sets of 8 to 12 reps with an 8- to 12-pound dumbbell*

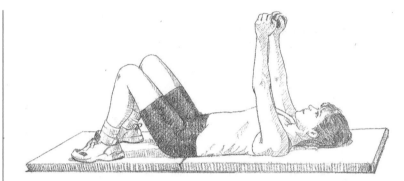

STEP 1: Lie face-up on a mat with your feet flat on the floor, about hip-width apart. Bend your knees so they point up to the ceiling, keeping your lower back pressed against the floor. Hold the dumbbell sideways so that one knob is in each hand. Extend your arms straight up, making sure your elbows aren't locked and your wrists, elbows, and shoulders are aligned.

Key things to remember
• Don't lock elbows
• Press lower back against floor
• Place feet hip-width apart
• Align wrists, elbows, and shoulders

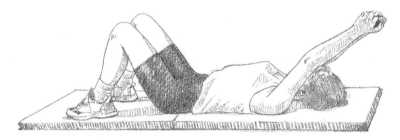

STEP 2: Exhale and keep your arms straight as you take four counts to slowly lower the dumbbell a little farther than halfway to the floor. Hold the position for one count, then inhale as you take two counts to slowly raise the dumbbell back to the starting position. Repeat.

Key things to remember

- Lower dumbbell more than halfway to floor
- Press lower back against floor
- Relax head and neck

Listen to Your Body

If you feel a strain in your neck or shoulders when you do the pullover, you're either lowering the dumbbell too far toward the floor or you're using a weight that's too heavy. "Focus on moving your arm from the shoulder, making sure there's no tension in your neck," says exercise physiologist Jennifer Layne. If you still feel tension, you may want to try doing the move without a dumbbell and focusing on keeping your back flat.

THE EXERCISES

The Swan

▶ **WHAT IT DOES**
Works the muscles in your upper back that give you good posture

▶ **GO FOR YOUR GOAL**
Drop a Dress Size: *6 to 8 reps on each side*

Shape Up: *8 to 12 reps on each side*

Maintain: *12 to 16 reps on each side*

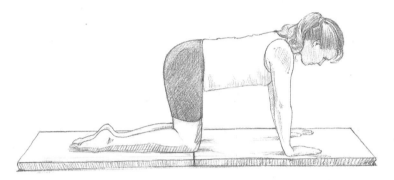

STEP 1: Start on all fours on a mat, with your hands directly under your shoulders and your knees directly under your hips. Keep your back straight and your eyes looking down at the floor. Point your toes and avoid locking your elbows.

Key things to remember
• Look down
• Align neck with spine
• Align hips with knees
• Align shoulders with wrists

• Keep back flat
• Don't lock elbows
• Point toes

LISTEN TO YOUR BODY

One of the most common errors with the swan exercise is sticking your chin out a bit so that your head tilts back and your neck shortens. "You want to make sure you're looking down at the floor throughout the move, with your chin tucked in slightly in most of the positions," says certified personal trainer Karen Andes. "When you're fully extending your arm and leg, keep your neck long and straight, as if you could balance a teacup on it."

You should also keep in mind that this dance exercise is a fluid movement, so you should not stop to hold each position. When your arm and leg are fully extended, you want to really reach in opposite directions with your arm and leg so you feel a good stretch in your back and shoulder.

If you find this exercise to be tough on your supporting knee, try using a pillow to cushion the joint, Andes suggests.

STEP 2: To move into the second position, pull in your stomach as you round your back and lift your right arm and left leg a few inches off the floor. Your right arm should be rounded, with elegant, extended fingers. Your leg should be bent at the knee so that your lower leg is parallel to the floor. As you round your back, your head will naturally tuck in toward your chest.

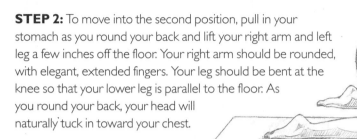

Key things to remember
- Pull stomach in
- Round back
- Drop head
- Round arm
- Point toes
- Lift knee toward chest

STEP 3: Continue contracting your abs as if you're pulling your belly button toward your spine. Extend your right arm and your left leg so that your arm is rounded, with your

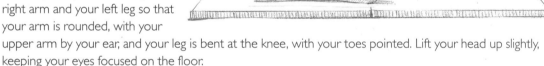

upper arm by your ear, and your leg is bent at the knee, with your toes pointed. Lift your head up slightly, keeping your eyes focused on the floor.

Key things to remember
- Extend leg
- Keep leg slightly bent
- Hold upper arm next to ear
- Lift head slightly

STEP 4: Fully extend your right arm and left leg so that they're straight and parallel with the floor. Lift your head back to its original position, with your neck in line with your spine and your eyes looking straight down. Your back should be flat like a tabletop.

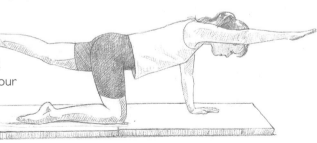

Key things to remember
- Flatten back
- Don't lock elbow
- Align neck with spine
- Fully extend leg
- Fully extend arm

(continued)

The Swan—Continued

▶ **TAKE IT
TO THE MAX**
You can make the swan exercise more difficult by strapping on some ankle weights. Just make sure you've mastered the move before you add weight, cautions certified personal trainer Karen Andes. "For this exercise, try using between 1 and 5 pounds."

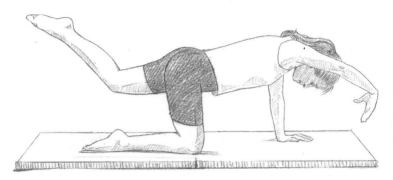

STEP 5: Round your right arm downward and bend your left knee so that you're in the same position as you were before you fully extended your arm and leg. Your back should be slightly rounded, with your head tucked downward a bit and your abs pulled in.

Key things to remember
- Round arm
- Round back
- Bend knee slightly
- Contract abs
- Tuck down head slightly

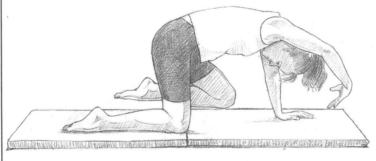

STEP 6: Bring your head, arm, and leg down and in toward your body as you round your back further and continue to contract your abs. This is the same position as the second one of this exercise. Then return to the starting position so that you're on all fours with your back flat and your neck in line with your spine.
Do your next repetition with your left arm and right leg. Continue alternating sides with each repetition.

Key things to remember
- Keep back rounded
- Tuck chin almost to chest
- Contract abs
- Hold lower leg parallel to floor
- Point toes

THE STRETCHES

Cat Stretch

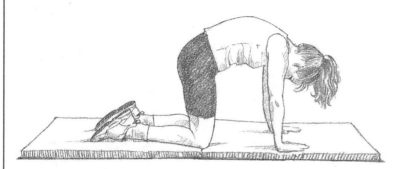

▶ WHAT IT DOES

Lengthens the muscles in your upper and middle back

▶ HOW TO DO IT

Start on all fours on a mat, with your hands directly under your shoulders and your knees directly under your hips. Pull in your stomach as you round your back. Your head will naturally drop down a bit, but you should avoid tucking your chin all the way to your chest. If you have knee problems or feel discomfort in your knees when you do this stretch, try putting a pillow under your knees.

Key things to remember

- Align knees with hips
- Align wrists with shoulders
- Round back
- Contract abs
- Drop head slightly

▶ DESKTOP TRAINER

Seated Cat Stretch

This stretch helps loosen the muscles in your back that tighten up when you sit for long periods, says exercise physiologist Jennifer Layne. Sit upright in your chair with your feet flat on the floor, about shoulder-width apart. Bend forward and round your back. Grab onto your shins, and hold the stretch for 30 seconds.

The Mind You've Thought About

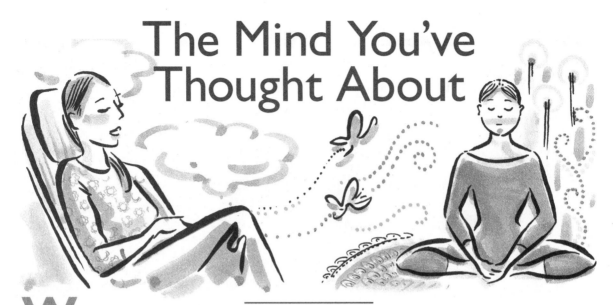

When the heaviest snowfall descends upon the surface of a placid lake, what do we hear?

Think.

We hear nothing. Only the most profound silence. The quiet calmness of the water remains undisturbed by the falling snow.

If only our minds, our spirits, were like that. If only we could remain calm and centered and undisturbed under the stresses of job, marriage, children, and community that fall upon us. How wonderful to accept and absorb, with peace and serenity, all that happens to us.

What is the use, finally, of having a strong, healthy body without a calm, resilient spirit? Our health and beauty depend on both.

Yet it sometimes seems that a healthy mind is the last thing that the world wants for us. As women, we find ourselves constantly on call to tend to the needs of everyone else. We nurse, we nurture, we give support. And we do it with love. We give of ourselves until it feels as if there's nothing left to give. At those times, we can easily find ourselves ignoring our bodies' calls for physical rest and pushing past our psyches' limits to the very brink of stress-

induced frenzy. Or we can simply make ourselves sick.

It's at those very times when we need to be like a perfectly peaceful lake under a falling snow. And with practice, we can.

Movement

In the West, we are only now beginning to catch up to what Eastern traditions have known for ages: The body and the mind are mated. And that means that, for better or for worse, what affects one inevitably affects the other.

Stress and anxiety are excellent examples. What woman alive hasn't experienced a major headache after a day of deadlines or demanding family errands? And we all know how a drawn-out illness can sap the spirit.

Rather than trying to forcibly bring the body or mind under control, the secret to beating stress lies in linking the two. The East has the right idea—Asian traditions of movement like tai chi, yoga, and aikido aren't simply ways to get into shape. Their precise, subtle motions are meant to ease the soul as well as the body.

"Movement and exercise can enhance the flow of energy in the body," says Margaret Matsumoto, senior instructor at the School of Tai Chi Chuan in Manhattan. "Movement integrates and balances the body parts with each other and with the mind."

To better understand what she means, try these special techniques from tai chi and yoga, and learn what it's like to move into a stress-free space.

Tai chi body-awareness exercise. "As two-legged creatures, we tend to stand double-weighted, utilizing only half of each leg's capacity," says Matsumoto. To help balance your body—and remain balanced and adaptable in any situation—you need to develop each leg to 100 percent of its capacity.

Stand with your feet hip-width apart and your knees relaxed. Allow your arms to float, draped lightly away from the sides of your body. Slowly begin to shift your weight back and forth, from one leg to the other, keeping your feet firmly on the floor and your spine straight. Notice if you feel strong in one leg or tired or off-balance.

Standing with our weight centered over one leg is foreign to most of us. Take your time to get accustomed to it as you learn to use each leg to its full capacity. "Let your body do the thinking," advises Matsumoto. Continue the exercise for at least 5 minutes.

Yoga mudra. Yoga asanas, or poses, are intended to increase flexi-

WOMAN TO WOMAN
Touched by a Therapist

Melody Maulding, a 38-year-old full-time mother and wife from the Seattle-Tacoma area of Washington, is plenty busy raising three girls. One is entering her teens, and the two others are 10-year-old twins with developmental challenges. The last thing that Melody needs is back pain, but that's exactly what she had until she put her mind and a therapist's hands to work.

It started 15 years ago when I received an injury to my lower back and sciatic nerves that resulted in chronic back pain and headaches.

I tried everything—physical therapy, massage, pain pills, muscle relaxants, and anti-inflammatories. I was beginning to feel that there was no relief in sight. Then, I went to see Andrea Gordon, M.D., a family-practice physician who is also a clinical assistant professor of family medicine at the University of Washington in Seattle.

When Dr. Gordon first suggested therapeutic touch, I was skeptical. I had heard of it before, when I worked in a hospital's oncology unit. When a physician administers therapeutic touch, she moves her hands above the patient's skin in order to manipulate the energy field, which is supposed to promote physical and mental healing. But I considered it one of those mind-over-matter things that wouldn't help. Still, I consented, figuring, "What could it hurt?"

I was enlightened from the very first session. I sat there with my eyes closed while Dr. Gordon asked me to focus, breathe, and visualize my pain. I could feel the static as she passed her hand above my body. I soon began to visualize vivid colors and strange formations in the areas of my pain.

Dr. Gordon told me to ask these parts of me what they needed in order for the pain to release its hold on me. As strange as it sounds, I could hear them answer. The pain lessened and the tension decreased.

I still use the visualization and relaxation techniques today. The main thing that I've learned is how important it is to take time out to focus, breathe, and relax. Therapeutic touch is not a cure; it's a tool. But now I can have some control of the pain's effect on my life.

THE SCENTS OF SERENITY
Aromatherapy to Alleviate Anxiety

Everything old is new again. While aromatherapy is the hottest thing to hit drugstore shelves in recent years, the practice has actually been around for ages.

To ease mild anxiety or work toward easing agitation or irritability, certain essential oils are more effective than others, says Mindy Green, professional member of the American Herbalists Guild, director of educational services at the Herb Research Foundation in Boulder, Colorado, and coauthor of *Aromatherapy: A Complete Guide to the Healing Art.* Use the following oils regularly to get the best results. And feel free to mix and match scents with delivery techniques. Just make sure never to ingest essential oils or apply them directly to your skin in their undiluted form.

Lavender. Lavender is the universal oil for aromatherapy, says Green. It's safe and effective for treating a wide variety of problems, and "it's the rare person who doesn't like the odor," she says.

Add 5 to 8 drops of essential oil directly to a full bathtub of warm water. Or mix the same amount of lavender oil with a teaspoon of vegetable oil or shampoo, shake well, then add that mixture to the bathwater.

Neroli or petitgrain. Neroli oil comes from the flower of the exotic bitter-orange plant. Petitgrain oil, from the leaves and stems of the same plant, resembles neroli in scent and action but is less expensive.

Try a neroli or petitgrain mist for stress-induced insomnia. Add 5 to 8 drops of essential oil to a 2- to 3-ounce spray bottle of water, then mist your face and your body.

Marjoram. The essential oil of this herb is an excellent calmer as well as an antispasmodic. Try it along with a massage to treat muscle tension, headaches, or pain in your shoulders or back—classic signs of stress.

Add 10 drops of marjoram essential oil to 1 ounce of unscented body lotion to create a 2-percent dilution. Use the lotion liberally to knead and unkink tight muscles; or simply use it daily as a total-body, sense-soothing treat.

bility. But they are also meant to help you transcend mere physical existence by bringing your body and mind into harmony. One asana, in particular, called yoga mudra, can help to clear your mind of stress, according to Nora Anderson, yoga instructor, exercise physiologist, and president of the American Aerobic Association/International Sports Medicine Association in New Hope, Pennsylvania. Yoga mudra increases bloodflow to your brain and soothes your nervous system while it relaxes your muscles and improves flexibility in your hips and lower spine.

Remove your shoes, and kneel on a mat. Then sit back on your heels. If your buttocks don't easily reach your heels, use a pillow or folded blanket to bridge the space. You should be able to sit comfortably in this position. Reach your arms behind your body and clasp your hands together.

Exhale through your mouth as you bend forward toward the floor, leading with your chin, Anderson says. Let your arms raise up toward your head. Hold the position at a comfortable stretch for a count of 10, then inhale through your nose as you slowly raise yourself back into a sitting position. Briefly pause in the sitting position, then exhale through your mouth as you release your hands, let your arms come forward, and gently rest on your knees.

Repeat the above steps three times, Anderson suggests. Then carefully stand up. You can perform yoga mudra as often as once a day for the most mind-clearing benefits.

Breath

Inhale. Exhale. Inhale. Exhale.

Breathing is something that you probably don't think about much. That's because respiration is often (but not always, as we'll see) governed by the autonomic nervous system. When you're sleeping or having a conversation, for example, breathing is automatic and unnoticed.

At other times, breathing makes its presence felt by becoming tangibly out of control. Think of moments when your breathing becomes constricted, shallow, difficult, or impossible. Like during an asthma or panic attack. Or when choking sobs overtake you at a moment of grief. During times of stress, breathing changes—and not for the better. "It's a continuous feedback loop," says Matsumoto. "Anxiety can cause irregular breathing, but irregular breathing can also cause a feeling of anxiety."

Thankfully, the opposite is also true. When you switch over to your voluntary nervous system and take conscious control of your breath, wonderful things happen. "Breathing can be magical," says Matsumoto. "Properly done, it induces relaxation very quickly."

Try this right now: Inhale deeply through your nose to a count of four. Then slowly exhale through the mouth for twice as long—to a count of eight. Do it again. And once more.

There. After only three deep breaths, you

THE *KI* TO INNER PEACE

Ki, chi, qi, and *prana* are all words that describe the same phenomenon. According to practitioners of the Eastern arts of tai chi, aikido, and yoga, *ki* (pronounced "kee") and all of its synonyms describe your vitality, your life force, the energy you have coursing through your body. *Ki* is an intangible thing that your living, breathing body and striving, yearning soul gather from the universe.

The concept of *ki* can be hard to grasp. But getting a hold on this esoteric issue can be beneficial, especially to women, says Margaret Matsumoto, senior instructor at the School of Tai Chi Chuan in Manhattan. "Often, women burn their energy without getting anything back. For example, we may talk or worry excessively." Developing *ki,* instead of depleting it, can help women get in touch with their natural resources and deal with stress effectively, rather than burning out, she explains.

Cultivating *ki* is the main focus of many martial arts, such as tai chi and aikido. Other physical activities, like swimming or even running, can boost *ki* to some degree as well. But proper *ki* development involves your mind and spirit as well as your body, says Matsumoto. Here are some additional ways to foster *ki* abundance throughout your day:

- Eat fresh foods that are close to their natural state, such as fruits and whole grains.

- Honor tiredness by getting enough sleep each night; get extra rest when appropriate.

- Set aside a period of quiet, still time for meditation on a daily basis.

should feel noticeably different. Looser in your muscles, clearer in your head. This is in contrast to how most of us usually breathe. Intentionally slowing your breath down, deepening your inhalations, and drawing out your exhalations can have a profound effect. "When you choose to make your breath peaceful and rhythmic, it has a clearing, calming effect on both your body and your mind," says Anderson.

The discipline of yoga includes special breathing exercises called *pranayama*, which means "control of the vital life force." Some *pranayama* exercises involve breathing through alternating nostrils or retaining the breath for long periods of time. But you don't have to get complex to use your breath to your best advantage. Try this simple-but-effective yogic breathing technique, recommends Anderson.

The belly breath. You can practice this deep-breathing technique either seated comfortably in a chair or lying on your back on a mat or carpeted floor. Close your eyes and relax your body. Touch your palms to either side of your torso for a moment. Use your fingers and thumbs to gently feel the size and shape of your ribcage. "This will give you a sense of just how far down into the body your lungs actually extend, how large they actually are," says Anderson.

Relax one hand down beside your body, and place your other hand, palm down, on your lower abdomen just below your navel. As you inhale, visualize your belly as a big balloon, and allow it to press against your hand as it inflates. When you exhale, picture the imaginary balloon completely deflating as your belly sinks back toward your spine.

Five minutes or more of deep breathing can make a big difference at the end of a stressful day.

Stillness

Meditation is sort of like sleep. Like slumber, it is a natural, restoring state. In spite of science's great advances,

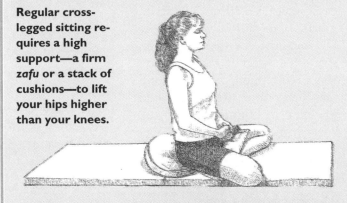

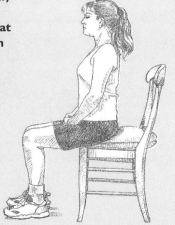

When doing *zazen* in a chair, sit on the edge of the seat and be sure your feet are flat on the ground. A pillow can be used to support your lower back.

Once you have established a comfortable position, rest your hands gently in your lap, the fingers of one hand gently cupped and cradled in the palm of the other. Then let your attention settle within the confines of your own body. "In Zen meditation, we try to let go of our thinking minds and bring our awareness to our bodies," says Phelan. "There's no special emphasis on breathing in a particular way, but just on breathing naturally."

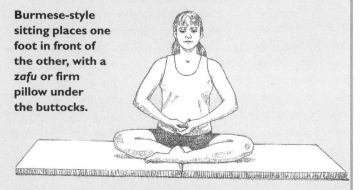

Burmese-style sitting places one foot in front of the other, with a *zafu* or firm pillow under the buttocks.

To help keep your mind clear and focused on the moment, try the technique of counting each breath. Without forcing or changing your pattern of breathing, notice each inhalation, then silently count each exhalation. Continue until you've numbered 10 exhalations. Then begin again.

How long you sit is up to you, Phelan says. The real emphasis should be placed on sitting *zazen* regularly.

both sleep and meditation remain a bit of a mystery. And, perhaps most intriguingly, just like sleeping, meditation is a do-it-yourself venture.

The catch is that meditation—or a good night's sleep, for that matter—can't be won by brute force. Struggling to silence the 101 thoughts plaguing your peace of mind only stands to make things worse. "Making a mental effort to quiet your mind is in itself another thought, another disturbance," says Ginny Whitelaw, Ph.D., chief instructor of aikido and Zen at the Atlanta Center for Zen and the Arts and author of *Body Learning: How the Mind Learns from the Body*.

The best way to quiet your mind is to first quiet your body. "You have to use the body-mind connection as a tool," says Dr. Whitelaw. Settling down physically—finding a quiet place to be still, either lying down or sitting upright—allows your mind to slow down as well.

Think of the energy in your body as a thermometer. When you are excited, you are literally "hot-headed," says Dr. Whitelaw. Your energy fills your mind. Bringing your energy level down into your body, into a place in your abdomen called the *hara* in Japanese, has a stabilizing and quieting effect. "It's the difference between being riled up and settled down," she says.

Savasana (corpse pose). Meditation is commonly done in a cross-legged seated position. But the supine yoga pose called *savasana* is an excellent way to get a feel for the effect that quieting your body has on stilling your mind.

REAL-LIFE SCENARIO

She Needs to Stress De-Stressing

Isabel, after 15 years of being a stay-at-home mom, went back to school, got her master's, then landed herself a high-powered job with a management-consulting firm. She makes a great salary and travels to interesting places all over the world. With all this, she also maintains a loving relationship with her husband and her grown son and daughter. The only problem is that with so many responsibilities, her stress levels are through the roof. To deal with them, she religiously exercises every other day. She jumps rope to get her wind up, then she pumps iron. In fact, she pumps heavy iron, and with a vengeance, as if she were getting even with someone she doesn't like. Yet, with all that exercising, her shoulders are tense and raised, and she feels as if she lives life in a pressure cooker. What can she do?

Isabel is doing plenty already—except dealing with the overabundance of stress in her life. Like a lot of women, she mistakenly assumes that a good, hard bout of exercise will reduce stress. But exercise *is* stress. And Isabel's "with-a-vengeance" approach to it makes resistance training just one more source of stress in her already stressful life.

It may sound odd that something as healthy as resistance training can be a source of stress. But it's not odd at all if you keep in mind that stress is not in and of itself a bad thing. There are lots of good sources of stress, such as Isabel's loving relationship with her husband or continued contact with her grown children. As far as her body is concerned, stress is stress—neither positive nor negative. It's the accumulation of it to unmanageable levels that causes problems.

By all means, Isabel should continue her exercise, but to deal with her stress levels she should take advantage of stress-management techniques such as meditation, yoga, and breathing exercises. At the same time, she should look around to see what stressors in her life—mental and physical—she could do without. Then she should get rid of them.

Expert Consulted
Nan Kathryn Fuchs, Ph.D.
Nutritionist
Sebastopol, California

This yoga position, often considered one of the most difficult to master, doesn't involve twisting, turning, balancing, or bending your back. All that it requires is complete and total relaxation of every single muscle in your body.

Lie on your back on a mat, on a carpeted floor, or even on the top of your bed. Separate your legs so your ankles are about 18-inches apart, and let your feet gently fall out to the sides. Let your arms rest about 6 inches from the sides of your body, with your palms facing up. Be sure that your body is symmetrical in this position. Then close your eyes and bring your attention to your breathing.

Let gravity pull the weight of your body toward the floor. Breathe slowly and deeply, allowing your abdomen to swell with each inhalation. Scan your body for tension, letting go and relaxing further and further. Remain in this pose for as long as is comfortable. When you're ready to come out of *savasana*, slowly roll onto your right side, then use your hands to gradually push yourself up to a sitting position.

Practicing *savasana* just once will leave your mind refreshingly calm and clear, and your muscles more relaxed than they've been in ages. When practiced more often—daily, if possible—the peace that you cultivate in this posture will overflow into the rest of your hours and become a background for the activity of your daily life, says Dr. Whitelaw.

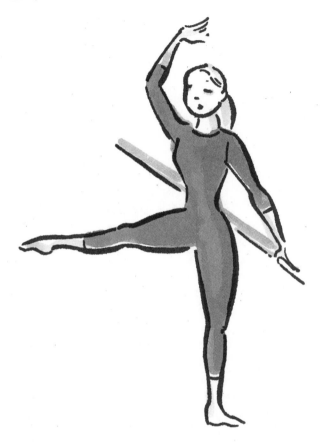

PART THREE

Exercising Options

Hey, What about Aerobics?

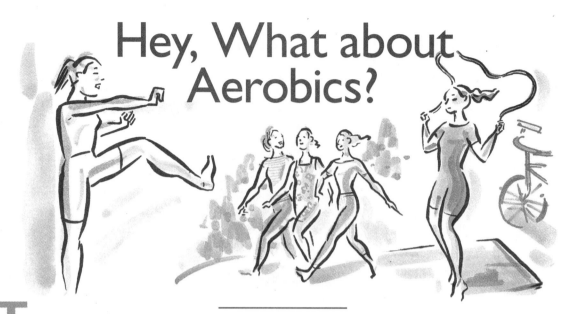

Talk about sacrilege. . . . How can we have gotten more than halfway through an exercise book without a walking, running, or Spinning program in sight?

Rest assured, it's not because aerobic exercise is anything less than it's cracked up to be. "For weight loss, endurance, and anything related to your heart, aerobic exercise is key," says Lisa Womack, associate director of the Cardiac Health and Fitness Memorial Gym at the University of Virginia in Charlottesville. "From a health standpoint, aerobics is very important."

In fact, do a little informal poll of your friends, and you'll probably see that most women prefer aerobic exercise to working with weights. But ask those same friends if they want taut and toned muscles, a well-sculpted figure, and a firmer-yet-feminine form from chin to shin, and you'll be hard-pressed to find a single one who'll say no. Aerobics, great as it is, will not accomplish those things for you. Toning exercises will.

This is not to say that you should toss out your aerobic exercise to concentrate on toning. Quite the contrary.

"Resistance training and aerobic training are two of the three components of total fitness," says Vicki Pierson, a certified personal trainer at the Fitness Jumpsite in Chatanooga, Tennessee. (Stretching exercise, for flexibility, is the third.) "They go hand in hand."

Doubling the Benefits

It's pretty obvious that jogging, biking, or jumping rope feels a lot different from working out with weights. Each will yield very different, though equally beneficial, results. That's because two radically different things are happening physiologically.

It comes down mostly to oxygen. When you do aerobic exercise, you increase your oxygen use over an extended period of time. Shorter bursts, or sprints, don't qualify. For energy, you burn calories.

Weight training, on the other hand, is anaerobic, meaning that your muscles use energy without primarily depending on oxygen. You may breathe harder for a quick period, but the object is to stress your muscles by making them work against resistance so they'll come back stronger.

Why do you need both types of exercise? Because you probably want to accomplish most or all of the following goals.

Lose body fat. Aerobic exercise is one of the best ways to do it, along with diet adjustments, of course. Building muscle mass through resistance training will bump up your resting metabolic rate, meaning that you'll burn more calories throughout the day even when you're not exercising. But that works only to support or help maintain your weight-loss efforts. "You're not going to see a big difference, either way, in the scales from weight training alone," says Womack.

Get toned. Here's where resistance training does the job and where aerobic training doesn't. "Regular resistance training will make your muscles denser so that you look better," says Priscilla Clarkson, Ph.D., professor and associate dean of the department of exercise science at the University of Massachusetts School of Public Health and Health Sciences in Amherst. "They'll become firm rather than flabby, which is often a concern in areas like the backs of your arms and your stomach."

Build endurance. Aerobic work recruits the muscle fibers that specialize in endurance much more than resistance training does. So it makes perfect sense that aerobic exercise is the one that will help you enjoy those long hikes or bike rides.

Get stronger. Appearance aside, strength training will make you stronger. Aerobics, on the

WHAT'S UP WITH THIS?

Electrical Muscle Stimulation

It has been advertised as the way to tone your trouble spots without breaking a sweat. Just hook yourself up to some pricey device, say its distributors, and an electrical impulse travels to your muscle, forcing it to contract and relax as it would during exercise.

Can you really tone your tummy while relaxing in a La-Z-Boy?

Don't put down your dumbbells just yet, says Margareta Nordin, D.Sc., a physical therapist and director of the Occupational Industrial Orthopedic Center Hospital for Joint Diseases at New York University Medical Center in New York City. "For normal, healthy people, electrical muscle stimulation is merely a gimmick," she says.

First of all, your muscles do not contract to the degree that they would if you were doing exercises. You also miss out on moving your body through it's range of motion, one of the important benefits of exercise. Nor do you reap any of the cardiovascular benefits that you get from brisk walking or other aerobic activities. Not to mention that you have about 430 voluntary muscles in your body, and it would be nearly impossible to electrically stimulate all of them, Dr. Nordin says.

That's not to say that electrical muscle stimulation doesn't have any practical uses. Physical therapists use it as part of rehabilitation for patients who've had knee surgery, for example, and to help people who are paralyzed maintain muscle tone and elasticity.

other hand, won't do much to help you lift that growing 3-year-old or carry heavy stuff without having to ask for help.

Get a strong heart. This is a job for aerobics. It's your heart that has to pump all of that oxygen to your muscles via your bloodstream when you're doing your aerobic work. That's why your heart rate goes up. And that's why aerobic exercise is a proven strengthener of your cardiovascular system and a risk reducer for heart disease.

Spot train. It bears repeating: Neither aerobic exercise nor diets can target fat in any one body part for elimination. For that matter, neither can resistance training. "If you could spot reduce, everyone who chewed gum would have a skinny face," Womack says. But what resistance training *can* do—and aerobics can't—is target body parts for muscle toning. When you do toning exercises, you can say, "I'm going to work on my thighs today." Not so with aerobics.

Boost your bones. The two can team up to help prevent osteoporosis or mitigate its effects. Weight-bearing aerobic exercises such as running (but not swimming or cycling) help strengthen your bones. So does weight training, which also builds your strength to help prevent the falls that so often lead to broken bones for women with osteoporosis. "The research is pretty clear that the best exercise program for osteoporosis is going to combine weight-bearing aerobic exercise with weight training," Dr. Clarkson says.

Shaky Marriages

Once you realize the complementary benefits of aerobic exercise and toning, the search is on for a plan for doing both. You're now a candidate for cross-training, that multipurpose word for, basically, doing more than one kind of exercise. There are some good ways to do it and some not-so-good ways. Here are the options.

Getting muscle work from the aerobic exercise itself. Even "pure" aerobic exercises require some muscle work, although the "resis-

WOMEN ASK WHY

Why don't I ever hear about calisthenics anymore?

It's pretty easy to have mixed feelings about calisthenics. On the one hand, the word comes from two Greek roots meaning "beauty" and "strength"—two qualities that are certainly worth saving from extinction. On the other, it will forever be associated with that sadistic physical-education teacher you had in high school. No wonder it's an endangered exercise species.

Calisthenics usually refers to an exercise routine that you do without weights or any other equipment. Well-known calisthenics movements include pushups, situps, jumping jacks, running in place, and leg raises.

You can see from that partial list that calisthenics haven't entirely disappeared. The "leg work" that is tacked on to many aerobics classes is a lot like calisthenics. In any weight-training routine, workouts for your midsection will consist mostly of crunches and similar exercises. And pushups are still considered a pretty good upper-body strengthener.

Some traditional calisthenics movements, however, have turned out to do more harm than good, deep knee bends

tance" that your muscles are working against may be only gravity or water. There is some toning benefit in this, as many aerobics enthusiasts will tell you. But for a number of reasons, those benefits are very limited, experts agree.

First of all, most of the more popular aerobic exercises—walking or running, cycling, stairclimbing, and aerobics classes—tax your leg muscles and little else. That hardly squares with your overall toning goals. "Most aerobics work only the lower-body muscles," Dr. Clarkson says. "But it's in the upper body where most women aren't very strong and want more definition."

being a prime example. That's one reason for calisthenics' fade. Another is those negative associations. Yet another is that—let's face it—calisthenics are boring. And if you really want to be cynical, you can blame their demise on the fact that it's pretty hard to sell merchandise around such an equipment-free, no-frills mode of exercise.

But the main reason that you don't hear too much about calisthenics these days is that we've found better ways of getting fit. In the last few decades, new knowledge about aerobic exercise has pushed jumping jacks into dinosaur land. More important (since strength and toning is the main goal of calisthenics), resistance training has been shown to get results more quickly, more thoroughly, and more easily than any calisthenics routine. Weights let you adjust the resistance so you can make steady progress. Weights also let you concentrate on individual muscles in a way that calisthenics can't.

And, yes, weight training is a lot more fun.

Expert Consulted
Lisa Womack
Associate director of the Cardiac Health and
    Fitness Memorial Gym
University of Virginia
Charlottesville

Even the more "full-body" aerobic workouts—rowing, swimming, and cross-country skiing—are far from ideal for toning purposes. You're still using only specific muscles, instead of hitting all of them as you would in a good resistance-training workout. More important, you're using them in a different way—calling on their endurance capacity, rather than directly improving their absolute strength as you do with resistance training.

Adding weights to your aerobic workout. It's a common sight: eager exercisers using hand weights while they walk in the park, ride their exercise bikes (not real ones on a bike path, hopefully), or do aerobics in front of a video. Bad

idea, say the experts. Essentially, you're sacrificing some of the aerobic effect for a sloppy and incomplete weight workout. Besides, it's dangerous.

"When you use hand weights, you usually end up slowing down your pace, so using the weights will typically make the aerobic exercise easier, not harder," Womack says. "Yet the injury rate goes up dramatically because carrying weights in your hands tends to throw off your posture and overstress your joints."

Using strap-on ankle weights during aerobics is even worse, for the same reasons. "They're a big no-no," Pierson says.

Circuit training with weights. Remember when weight machines got real popular in the 1980s? With them came the notion of circuit training. In this case, that means getting an aerobic workout while you weight train by moving promptly from machine to machine, thus keeping your heart rate up.

But this is not your best bet. The aerobic effect may not be all that it's said to be, according to Womack. "There's a nice linear relationship between heart rate and oxygen consumption for exercises like walking or biking, but it doesn't exist with weight training," she says. "Though your heart rate stays elevated, your oxygen consumption levels are about equal to a very moderate walk."

Besides, haste makes waste. "Circuit training works on the premise that you're trying to do things fast to keep your heart rate up," Womack says. "So you tend to have sloppy form and not go through the entire range of motion."

Circuit training with aerobics and weights. The idea here is to alternate true aerobic work

---

WHAT'S UP WITH THIS?

Oxycise!

If you do aerobic exercise, you probably perform the two-fingered neck press on occasion to check your heart rate. But in reality, it's the amount of oxygen being delivered to your cells that matters; your heart rate is just a convenient way of measuring, since it corresponds to oxygen intake.

So if the key to calorie burning is oxygen, why bother with exercise? Why not just breathe in more oxygen while you're sitting down? That's precisely the idea behind Oxycise!, a 15-minute breathing routine that is available on video. The system claims to deliver the weight-loss benefits of aerobic exercise, without the impact.

Breathing techniques such as those practiced in yoga have a long history of health benefits, but Oxycise! breathing is different, according to founder Jill Johnson. "It's very powerful, rather than relaxing and meditative," she says. "You pump it in and blow it out hard, as if you were running."

Oxycise! facilitates toning, too, says Johnson. "I have you lifting and tucking and tightening," she says. "There are so many things your body can do while you're breathing."

Needless to say, experts are not recommending that you abandon your tried-and-true resistance training and aerobics workouts for such alternative newcomers. But since Oxycise! uses no equipment, takes only 15 minutes, and doesn't even require you to stand up, you can give it a try while you're sitting around watching television. What the heck, we all have to breathe, don't we?

---

into 5- or 10-minute increments will still yield aerobic benefits. "For combining aerobics and strength training, this kind of circuit training is a better option," Pierson says.

Separate but Equal

The best strategy, by far, for getting both your aerobic and toning workouts is to separate them and give each the individual attention that it deserves. "Your best program will have focused aerobic time and focused weight-training time," Womack says. "Not both at once."

Does that sound overly time-consuming? It's not. There are lots of ways to satisfy both of your exercise needs, and one is surely right for you.

Switch excess aerobic days to toning. Are you one of those women who loves aerobics (and its results) so much that you do it five, six, or even seven times a week? Good for you, but chances are, you'd benefit more by replacing two of those days with a strength-training workout. You'll get the best of both with no additional time commitment. "For most women, 3 or 4 days of aerobics and 2 or 3 days of strength training are plenty," Pierson says.

Switch excess toning days to aerobics. If you like your weight work so much that you find yourself doing all of your strength exercises almost every day, you're probably not getting the benefits that you should—and not leaving yourself some free days for aerobics. "You need to wait at least 48 hours between workouts since

---

with your weight work. "You may use the treadmill for 10 minutes and then work on one body part with weights," Pierson says. "Then maybe cycle for 10 minutes before you work another body part. And so on."

Of course, at home you may not have the luxury of a variety of aerobic machines. But splitting up even one type of aerobic exercise

your muscles are repairing themselves," Pierson says. "So you can do aerobics one day and strength training the next." Three days a week, then, is pretty much the max for full-body weight sessions, leaving 4 days open for nothing but aerobics.

Use your time wisely. You may prefer to do your aerobic and toning work on the same days. But you find that after an hour of working with weights, you have little time and even less desire to do your half-hour of aerobics. The solution is to streamline your toning time. "You don't need to spend an hour doing strength training to hit all the major muscle groups," Pierson says. "Instead, do a 5- to 10-minute warmup, such as walking in place, then spend an efficient 30 minutes with the weights and the other 30 minutes doing aerobics. Don't forget to stretch your muscles after the aerobics."

Be a one-timer. Free up time and energy for same-day aerobicizing by doing one set of each strength-training exercise instead of two, Womack suggests. In other words, instead of doing a dumbbell movement 8 times (or 10, or 12, or whatever), then resting, then doing it 8 more times, just do it the first 8 times and move on. Voilà! You've cut your toning time in half without sacrificing benefits. For a general fitness population, one set of 10 repetitions for each weight-training exercise is almost, although not quite, as good as two, Womack says. "That makes a difference if you're time-pressed."

WHAT'S UP WITH THIS?

The Lama Exercise

Scan the Internet for "aging and exercise," and sooner or later, you're bound to come across the instructions for "the Lama exercise," reputedly discovered in the early part of this century in a Tibetan monastery by a Briton seeking the fountain of youth.

The exercise includes five steps. The first is simply spinning with your arms outstretched. The next four are poses that all have a counterpart in yoga.

The individual movements require instructions and guidance, says Theresa Rowland, director and recreational therapist at Studio Yoga in Madison, New Jersey. The last three movements involve back bends, difficult poses that require a great deal of strength and flexibility, she says. The first of the backward-bending movements requires an open chest and strong spinal muscles in order to not injure your neck and lower back. The second backward movement is presented without the necessary support from the shoulder blades to open the chest and keep the shoulders in alignment. Part of the second and all of the third backward bends are done with your weight on your hands, which requires an understanding about extending and not collapsing your wrists.

The leg lifts may aggravate lower-back and neck injuries and ovarian cysts, Rowland continues.

"I am always interested to learn about movement sequences that have been practiced for centuries, sequences that have been inspirational and beneficial over time," says Rowland. "This is what I find lacking in this case. The Internet is not being used properly to introduce a sequence that must have much more depth than is being presented." In fact, these poses are quite easily done incorrectly, she says, and are best learned with a bona fide yoga instructor.

Get intense. Researchers have come up with another way to help you get your toning and aerobic work done on the same day and still have time for a life. "Basically, make time for your weights by cutting your aerobic time while bumping up the intensity," says Womack. That works because, as it turns out, 20 to 30 minutes at higher levels is more effective than 40 to 50 minutes of more moderate aerobic effort. "A lot of people don't know this because there's always been that myth that you had to go slow and long," Womack says. "But you actually burn more fat in the long run with a shorter, more intense bout of aerobic exercise."

There is one caveat, though. There are lots of medical reasons why more intensive aerobic work may not be right for you. Check with your doctor before turning up the intensity.

Spread it out. Having trouble fitting *any* half-hour block into your already full schedule?

Try a piecemeal approach. "We used to think that you had to exercise aerobically for a full 20 to 30 minutes at a time to get cardiovascular and other health benefits," says Karla A. Kubitz, Ph.D., assistant professor of kinesiology at Towson University in Maryland. "We now know that you still get benefits out of 5 minutes here, 5 minutes there, and 5 minutes somewhere else."

The same thing applies to your toning exercises. There's no need to work all of your muscles in one session, or even in 1 day. Six or seven 5-minute sessions spread over 3 days will meet your twice-a-week, work-every-body-part requirements. "Spreading it all out is one way of minimizing time problems," Dr. Kubitz says.

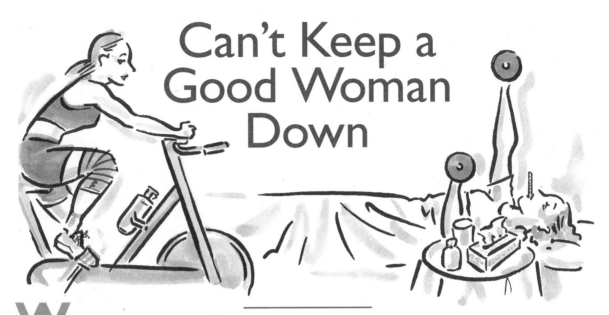

Can't Keep a Good Woman Down

When you're doing a squat, there's one sound—one feeling, actually—that you should fear, and it goes like this:

Pop!

It's often the first sign of an injury—in this case, an injury to the anterior cruciate ligament in your knee.

Sports- and exercise-related injuries can be frustrating, painful, and debilitating, and if you're not careful, far too easy to come by. Even though the light lifting and floor exercises that most women do are remarkably safe, we also have looser, less stable joints than men, which make us more likely to get hurt.

So what can we do to protect ourselves?

Know Your Enemy

Maybe because we don't show off so much, women seldom suffer acute injuries from toning exercises, even if we're doing resistance training. We don't heave around the kind of weight that, mishandled, can blow out a joint or rupture a disk. Instead, women may develop chronic injuries such as muscle strains, tendonitis, or bur-

sitis, which creep up on us over time because of poor form, says Karen Andes, author of several books on mind-body fitness and a certified personal trainer at Nautilus of Marin in San Rafael, California.

"The challenge," she says, "is distinguishing delayed-onset muscle soreness—'good pain,' which is uncomfortable but doesn't cause any permanent damage—from 'bad pain,' which may mean more serious problems such as tendinitis, ligament strain, or muscle tears."

Good pain is usually in the body of your muscles, the fleshy parts. It tends to happen on both sides of your body, come on slowly, and disappear quickly, Andes says. Bad pain—that is, injury—is usually on one side of your body, in a joint, or in your spine; and it tends to come on quickly and stick around. "Women can usually tell the difference between the two," she says.

Rest and ice are always appropriate if you develop pain. Stop using the muscle, and apply a bag of crushed ice, wrapped in a towel, if you like. Apply the ice for 10 to 15 minutes, then remove it for about a half-hour or so before applying it again as needed, says Michelle F.

Mottola, Ph.D., associate professor of anatomy and kinesiology and director of the exercise and pregnancy lab at the University of Western Ontario in London, Ontario. "Stop exercising immediately if you develop pain or discomfort. And seek medical advice immediately if your pain is severe; if it's accompanied by some other symptom, such as tingling; if you have swelling; if you can't move a joint; or if minor pain hasn't disappeared with a week or so of ice and rest.

"Make sure to see a doctor to find out what's wrong," Dr. Mottola says. Then, follow your physician's directions for recovery. A good physical-therapy program can help you get back on track fast, so you may want to ask your doctor for a referral.

Do No Harm

Injuries can happen anytime, but the first few weeks of any exercise program tend to be particularly risky, says Jean Reeve, Ph.D., a triathlete and associate professor of physical education at Southern Utah University in Cedar City. "Mentally, you may be raring to go; but at the same time, your body is just getting used to the idea of regular workouts," she says. "You need to slowly build up strength, especially around vulnerable knee and shoulder joints."

If you're overweight, you need to be especially careful about high-impact activities like running or jumping. They could hurt your joints.

And if you're out of shape overall, Dr. Reeve suggests that you may do better by initially steering clear of activities that require good balance and coordination, such as step aerobics.

REAL-LIFE SCENARIO

She Tried to Be One of the Guys

When Terri, 40, went looking for a health club to join, she drove right past any place that had plush rugs, pastel colors, or soft lighting. She'd heard that for great results, she'd be best off going to a no-frills gym where members preferred free weights to fancy machines and where trainers were tough, no-nonsense experts on getting into shape. She found what she was looking for: a gym where people, mostly guys, grunted and turned red while lifting gargantuan stacks of iron. It wasn't long before she found herself getting into the spirit of the place, spending more and more time there and lifting weight so heavy that it tested the limits of her strength. She pushed herself harder and harder, and she made rapid progress. Now, suddenly, she has begun to feel weaker. More tired. She always seems to have a head cold or a chest cold, and she has started getting muscle and tendon pulls. What's happening to her?

Terri is overtraining. In fact, Terri's picture could be on a poster warning about the dangers of overtraining. She's a classic example of a common problem among women who are highly motivated to shape up: They let their zeal take them in the wrong direction.

It's not the emphasis on free weights or the macho atmosphere of her gym that led Terri astray. If that's the kind of place where she feels inspired, she should go for it. But she's adapting her routine to her surroundings, rather than the other way around. That is, she's modeling her workout after guys who don't have her body, her goals, or her life. As a result, she's obviously lifting too much weight, she's probably lifting it too often, and chances are, she's not lifting it correctly.

"You're better off building up some muscle first with some light resistance training and stair-climbing," she says.

If you're already suffering from an injury, take heart. You don't have to mothball your entire workout. "You probably can continue to do certain exercises," Dr. Reeve says. "But you may

Here's why that matters: Our muscles don't grow firmer and stronger during the actual workout. That happens during the recovery period that follows, as they repair themselves from the stress of the weight lifting. Noticeable improvement is a cumulative process. If you try to shortcut it with too-heavy weights or too-short recovery periods, you compromise the results and leave yourself susceptible to the kinds of injuries that Terri has been going through.

Such overtraining can have more serious consequences than merely disappointing results. Terri has experienced some of them, like lingering fatigue, frequent colds, and those injuries. Add to the list sleep disturbances, an elevated resting heart rate, and depression. It's a good bet that none of these things were on Terri's list of goals when she started her training.

Now that Terri has experienced firsthand the perils of overtraining, she'll probably be willing to adjust her routine to avoid them. That means she should do each exercise with a weight that's challenging at 8 to 12 repetitions, rather than with one that's impossible at 6. She'll benefit more by concentrating on quality (good form) instead of quantity (too-frequent workouts). To keep improving, she should add weight little by little at her own pace, ignoring what the guys around her are doing. And she must make sure that she doesn't work the same muscle group 2 days in a row.

Expert Consulted
Renee Cloe
Certified personal trainer
Cofounder of the Fitness Jumpsite Web site

Get your doctor to sign off. If you are age 45 or older, or if you have back or joint problems, osteoarthritis, osteoporosis, high blood pressure, or any other kind of chronic medical problem that makes you wonder if it's safe to exercise, Dr. Reeve suggests that you clear your plans with your doctor first. The evaluation should include a treadmill stress test, which can detect serious coronary artery blockage, and blood pressure and cholesterol measurements. If necessary, your doctor can suggest activities that you need to avoid.

Start like a tortoise, not a hare. Begin with a routine that is suited to your level of fitness. "For people who haven't exercised in a long time, start slow and easy," says Dr. Mottola. You'll beef things up as you progress. Eventually, you'll get the weight up to the point where 16 reps leaves your muscles pretty much pooped out.

If you're using a toning videotape, select one that fits your fitness level. You can always add on to your collection as you progress.

Start Right, Stay Right

If you've never toned before, learn how to do it right. The placement of each body part counts. "If you actively engage your mind in what you are doing, you can develop a body sense that helps you prevent injuries," Andes says. "Good form is important. You should know what muscles you are working."

Here are some tips on form that will help to make your workouts safer.

Don't lock your joints. In other words, don't completely straighten out your arm or leg

need to avoid using your injured area, or use it less strenuously. A physical therapist can help you figure out what moves to avoid until you're healed, and what exercises may actually help your injury heal faster."

Here are some items to consider before you begin exercising.

at the end of an extension. Locking up "may allow the limb to 'rest' a bit, but it's very hard on your joints," Andes says. "Joint tissue is not flexible, so if you stress the joint by overstretching it, it doesn't snap back. You can easily stress your joints over time and not even realize it, because joint pain accumulates quietly."

If you are doing an arm curl, for instance, start with your elbow bent. Then, as you lower the dumbbell, straighten your arm, but don't lock your elbow—keep it just slightly bent and keep your wrist straight. If you are doing flies, keep both your elbows slightly bent and your wrists straight, as if your arms are hugging a barrel. "You may need to use a bit less weight when you unlock your joints, but you're working just as hard," Andes says.

Aim for smooth, slow moves. Don't rely on speed or momentum to raise or lower a weight or to move your body weight around, Andes says. "You shouldn't jerk to get a weight moving. If you need to do that, the weight is too much." Most toning classes are way too fast, Andes says. "We go incredibly slow, working 4 to 10 seconds for each repetition. And working that slow, people say, 'I can't believe how much I can get out of these little 5-pound dumbbells.'"

Going slow helps you to focus in on the muscle that you are intending to work, and to maintain good form, Andes says. "It lets you do things like keep your shoulders down and back, and keep your torso steady," she says.

WOMAN TO WOMAN
She Ignored the Pain—And Suffered More

When Patti Florey, 48, started working with weights 5 years ago, she was typical in every way. A busy educational consultant in Mount Pleasant, Texas, Patti found time to add some strength workouts to her aerobic exercise, working her muscles at home with simple equipment and a lot of enthusiasm. But in October of 1998, something decidedly untypical happened—she suffered a ligament injury in her shoulder as a result of her weight work. With much of her strength-training routine shut down as she recovered, Patti had time to ponder what had gone wrong.

Before I started strength training, I'd never touched a weight in my life. But I'd always been interested in health issues, so I knew that working with weights would help my shape and my bones. Above all, I was determined to do things correctly. I even hired a wonderful personal trainer to guide me.

I work a tremendous number of hours, in addition to having the usual family obligations. I was also taking care of my chronically ill mother at the time. Still, I was able to do my race walking five times a week and strength training three times a week, exercising alone at home, as I prefer to do.

Of all of the benefits that I got from strength training, the one that pleased and surprised me the most was how much relief it gave me from my lower-back pain. I've had chronic back pain since I was a teenager, and weight training is the only thing in all those years that's helped me. It was wonderful.

In a roundabout way, I think that my experience with back pain had something to do with my injury. In the fall of 1998, I realized that I'd reached a plateau in my training, so I decided to add more weight to my exercises. But I added too much weight too quickly.

Mind your wrists. Women can easily hurt their wrists if their forearm muscles aren't strong enough to allow them to keep their wrists in a neutral position, in line with their forearms.

My body began giving me warning signals in the form of pain, but I kept working through it. All my life, I'd had to overcome an aching back to get things done, so I'd developed a pretty high pain tolerance. Now, I was misapplying my feisty determination, and the result was a partially torn rotator cuff in my shoulder.

I've paid a high price for my stubbornness. For one thing, a torn rotator cuff hurts more than I ever thought it could. Also, since I can't work my upper body until I've recovered—unless I'm doing a recovery exercise that's been prescribed by my orthopedist—I've lost the gains that I'd worked for. I don't feel as strong, and I don't look as toned in my upper body anymore. Worst of all, my back pain has increased again since I had to stop my weight training.

This injury is discouraging, but I'm not at all disgusted with weight training. In fact, I'm still doing my lower-body routine while my shoulder is recovering. I'm eager to start the upper-body work again, but I know that this time I'll have to be more faithful to my vow to do things correctly.

For one thing, I'll have to be patient and not try to come back until I'm ready. Proper form is also important; my trainer thinks that I may have contributed to the injury by bringing my shoulders too far behind me in some of my weight exercises. I'll definitely have to be careful about the amount of weight that I use. It's not always easy to tell what's an acceptable challenge as opposed to an unacceptable risk. I guess I'll err on the side of caution.

And of course, I'm going to have to rein in my determination to work through pain. My high pain threshold has helped me in other areas of life, but it only caused me trouble in my weight training. It won't happen again.

whether holding on to weights or a machine. If your wrists cock back and you can't hold them straight, you may be putting too much weight on them.

Forearm strengthening is involved in most biceps and back exercises, Andes says.

Exercise opposites. People tend to take a two-dimensional approach to their bodies, Andes says. "They work the parts they can see in the mirror." This means that the back of the body—equally important in terms of strength, balance, and injury prevention—is often neglected.

Just about every muscle has an "opposing" muscle, and both need to be exercised, Andes says. So don't forget about the muscles behind your shoulders, called external rotators. Or your hamstrings, the muscles on the backs of your thighs that oppose your quadriceps. "A well-planned total-body program provides this balance," Andes says.

Shake it up every once in a while. Even the best-planned toning routines benefit from an occasional shake-up, says Andes. "Muscles don't take long to get accustomed to what you are doing, so if you find yourself in a cozy little routine, before long your muscles will plateau. You just won't get any stronger." Even something as simple as changing the angle of attack on a weight, upping the intensity of your routine, or using resistance bands instead of weights can upset your routine enough that your muscles will begin to respond again. You're working more efficiently, so you get stronger with less effort, and you're helping to prevent overuse injuries.

This creates numbness and tingling, the kind of symptoms that are associated with carpal tunnel syndrome, Andes says. Avoid bending your wrists, no matter what exercise you're doing—

HEAVY BREATHING: IF EXERCISE TAKES YOUR BREATH AWAY

If you hack, wheeze, or come up short on air while you're doing an aerobic exercise or even when you stop to rest, you could have exercise-induced asthma. "It's common, especially when you're pushing yourself so hard that you breath through your mouth, which dries out your airways," says Joanne Blessing-Moore, M.D., a physician in Palo Alto, California, and a member of the American College of Asthma and Allergy sports medicine committee. Dry air—hot or cold—only makes things worse. This is a very common problem and it should not limit exercise, Dr. Blessing-Moore says. Your best recourse: Before you exercise, use an inhaler to reduce airway reactivity.

Toning exercises aren't likely to bring on exercise-induced asthma, but if you cough, wheeze, or have a bitter or acid taste in your mouth when you do situps or work on a decline, caustic stomach acid may be seeping into your windpipe, Dr. Blessing-Moore says. Make sure you exercise on an empty stomach, she suggests, or avoid working flat or on a decline.

Stop before you run out of gas. Bodybuilders sometimes "take a set to failure," that is, they lift a weight until their muscles give out. True, this technique does build muscle mass. But, to avoid injury, beginners need to pay careful attention to fatigue, and back off or stop when muscle fatigue interferes with their ability to perform toning exercises correctly, Dr. Reeve says.

You're Supposed to Hurt, But How Much?

After a typical resistance-training session, you will become sore. And you *should* become sore.

You should feel good pain, or burn. "The technical word is *delayed-onset muscle soreness*, or DOMS," Dr. Reeve says. It simply feels like you have used your muscles. It sets in gradually, 24 to 72 hours after a workout session, then slowly dissipates. It's due to the process of tissue repair that goes on in muscles after a hard workout. Some DOMS is inevitable when you begin toning or resistance training.

Here are some tips to reduce DOMS.

Warm up before you start any kind of exercise. Before you even go near a dumbbell, a weight machine, or resistance bands, do aerobic exercises to raise your body temperature until you break into a light sweat. "Hop on a stairclimbing machine, stationary bike, or treadmill," Andes suggests. "Or if you're planning to work mostly your upper body, use a rowing machine." If you're planning to lift heavy to moderate weights, warm up by doing a set with lighter weights that allow you to easily move your limbs through their full range of motion.

Save your serious stretching for afterward. Toning exercises don't leave you feeling muscle-bound. Still, unless you stretch, over time your muscles will become contracted and you will feel stiff. Stretch when you're really warmed up, after exercise, targeting those muscles that you have hit hard with toning exercises—your hips, buttocks, thighs, and torso, Andes says.

Make rest as important as exercise. It's when they are rebuilding after the stress of resistance training that your muscles get firmed up and toned. If you don't give them the chance to recover, over time you will start to have chronic injuries and pain, Dr. Reeve says. Some people rest by varying toning exercises one day with walking, yoga, or swimming the next day. Others work certain parts of their bodies one day and other parts the next day, giving their muscles at least 48 hours of rest between strenuous sessions.

Too Sick to Exercise?

"When in doubt, do it." That's Dr. Reeve's advice. "If I'm not sick enough to know for sure that I can't exercise, I'll at least try it," she says.

For those of us not quite so driven, Dr. Reeve offers this advice: If you have a head cold, go ahead and exercise. It may even make you feel better. But if you have a fever or you have symptoms below the neck, lay off. In other words, don't exercise if you have chest congestion or the flu.

How about if you're just feeling sluggish? "It could be mental, and in that case, exercise may help," Dr. Reeve says. If so, you'll know because soon into your workout, you'll begin to perk up. Switching your workout to your most energetic time of day may help, too.

If you often feel too tired to exercise, it's time to see your doctor. Several common, easily treated women's health problems, such as iron deficiency, can cause fatigue.

CAN YOU TONE WHILE YOU'RE PREGNANT?

Your body may feel like it's been taken over by aliens, but that doesn't mean you can't stay in shape when you're expecting. One study found that women who exercised vigorously—burning more than 1,000 calories a week—were more likely to carry their babies to full term than women who exercised less. If you're having a normal, healthy pregnancy and have your doctor's okay to exercise, here's what to keep in mind, according to Yvonne S. Thornton, M.D., clinical professor of obstetrics and gynecology at the University of Medicine and Dentistry of New Jersey–New Jersey Medical School in Newark and director of the Perinatal Diagnostic Testing Center at Morristown Memorial Hospital in New Jersey.

- During your first trimester, stay cool when exercising. Drink plenty of water, wear cool clothing, and don't work out in too hot of an environment. High body temperature can adversely affect fetal development.

- After your first trimester, don't do any exercises that require you to lie flat on your back. They can decrease bloodflow to your uterus.

- You'll have less oxygen available for aerobic exercise during pregnancy, so modify the intensity of your routine accordingly. Specifically, says Dr. Thornton, exercise at no more than 60 to 70 percent of your target heart rate. For women ages 20 to 29, that's 135 to 150 beats per minute; for women ages 30 to 39, 130 to 145 beats per minute; and 125 to 140 beats per minute for women 40 to 49. You can wear a heart-rate monitor; or count your heartbeat for 10 seconds, then multiply by six.

- Don't do any exercises in which you could lose your balance, especially in your third trimester, says Michelle F. Mottola, Ph.D., associate professor of anatomy and kinesiology and director of the exercise and pregnancy lab at the University of Western Ontario in London, Ontario. At this point, you may find buoyant water aerobics the best way to stay fit without stressing your joints. Dr. Thornton believes that swimming and walking are the best overall exercises for pregnant women.

Toning Your Diet

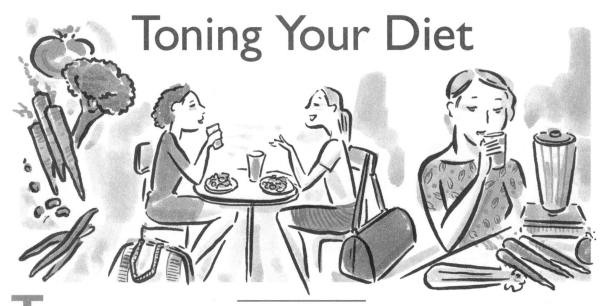

The average woman in America consumes more than 50 tons of food and 13,000 gallons of liquid over a lifetime. That translates into either a lot of fat or a lot of muscle, depending upon what we eat and how active we are. Most women would prefer having muscle, but is that what we usually end up with?

A lean, strong, toned body comes from proper care and feeding. That means combining the best exercises with the best foods, in the right amounts. It does not mean starving yourself and doing endless hours of aerobics to get your body fat down to dangerous levels.

The real trick is common sense and planning, based on some fundamental knowledge about eating, exercise, and your body.

Calories Count

After age 35, many of us put on weight we'd like to get rid of. Exercise can help us do that. But we also need to control our eating habits.

Maintaining or losing weight and staying in shape depends on energy balance. If you consume the same number of calories that you ex-

pend, your body maintains its weight. If you eat fewer calories than you burn, you lose weight. To lose 1 pound of body fat, you have to create a 3,500 calorie deficit. So if you cut your total daily caloric intake by 500 calories, you should be able to lose 1 pound a week

Just be careful not to cut your calories too low. You need to take in a minimum of 1,200 to 1,500 calories every day to keep your metabolism—your body's energy-burning mechanism—running at its optimum level. Eating less than that could actually make weight control more difficult.

"If you eat too few calories, after a while your body slows down its calorie-burning to adapt to the low fuel supply, and your weight loss may stop," says Stacey Whittle, R.D., a coauthor of *The Winning Edge of Sports Nutrition* and the nutritionist for the sports nutrition team at Florida Hospital in Orlando.

But there's a problem with depending on diet alone to shed pounds: When you lose weight, you lose more than fat.

"Up to 50 percent of the weight you lose may be muscle if you're not doing exercise that helps maintain muscle mass," says Nancy Clark, R.D., a nutritionist with Sports Medicine Brookline in Massachusetts and author of *Nancy Clark's Sports Nutrition Guidebook*. Muscle-building exercise can counter this effect somewhat, but not completely. "With exercise, the amount of muscle you lose may drop from one-half to about one-third of your total weight loss," she says. "So for every 2 pounds of fat you lose, you'll lose only 1 pound of muscle."

When you decide you've lost enough fat through exercise and changing your eating habits, your body will start to rebuild muscle, and the scale may go up a few pounds. Don't panic—it's not fat, Clark says. Having more muscle will do more than just make you stronger and improve your shape. It will also help you keep the fat off.

That's because each pound of muscle you have burns 40 to 50 calories a day. The more you have, the more you burn. "Just a couple of pounds of muscle can make a big difference in whether you can have a treat or two a day without gaining weight," says Clark. "In comparison, a pound of fat burns virtually no calories. It really is baggage."

Of course, you don't burn up or store as fat everything that comes into your body. You also need nutrients to build tissue, including muscle. That's where protein comes in.

Protein Power

Your body makes muscle from the protein you eat, not from carbohydrates or fats. Excess protein is

---

REAL-LIFE SCENARIO
Her Belly Is Getting Bigger, Not Smaller

At age 45, Melinda looked down one morning to put on her shoes and realized that she couldn't see her feet. Her belly was in the way. As a young woman, she had always thought that her slender, strong, flat midsection was one of her best features. But the tummy she had now was not only unflattering, it made her feel unhealthy. She immediately set out to get it under control. She remembered most of the stomach exercises she used to do for high school gymnastics, and she began doing them with a vengeance: crunches, leg raises, bicycles, twists. She was looking forward to buying smaller-size clothes within a few months, but the unthinkable has happened: She has found that her waist is getting bigger instead of smaller. She's horrified. What can she do?

Melinda is using the wrong tool for the job. Her midsection exercises are yielding results—namely, toned and stronger muscles under her tummy. But her belly is still big because the excess fat is still there. So she can crunch from now until her 50th high school reunion and never shrink her belly.

In fact, Melinda has discovered that her newly developed muscles have indeed grown a tad. This healthy growth would be contributing to her shapeliness and making her clothes fit better if it weren't buried under so much fat.

Also, Melinda may be eating even more than before, under the mistaken impression that she is "working off" those meals with crunches. But crunches—or any other strength-training exercise—don't burn as many calories as she needs to in order to lose weight. And those excess calories that have been stored as fat are what have caused her problem in the first place. If the excess keeps growing, so does her tummy.

The answer for her is a combination of aerobic exercise, such as walking, cycling, or swimming, and a better diet, along with her crunches and other abdominal work.

Expert Consulted
Jill Kanaley, Ph.D.
Assistant professor of exercise physiology
Syracuse University
New York

stored as fat, however. And research shows that Americans tend to eat too mush protein, according to Carla Wolper, R.D., a nutritionist at the Obesity Research Center at St. Luke's–Roosevelt Hospital Center in New York City. So turning that protein into muscle instead of letting it hang around as fat is yet another motivation to exercise.

Adequate protein intake for building muscle mass is about 0.7 gram of protein per pound of body weight a day, says Wolper. That's about twice the Recommended Dietary Allowance.

If you're more than 20 pounds overweight, calculate the amount of protein you need based on an ideal weight for your height. To figure out your ideal weight, figure in 100 pounds for the first 5 feet of height and 5 pounds an inch thereafter. For example, if you're 5 foot 6 inches, your ideal weight would be 130, give or take 10 percent, says Wolper.

To figure out how this translates into servings of food, use these figures.

- 7 grams of protein in 1 ounce of meat, chicken, fish (salmon or cod), lunchmeat (turkey), or low-fat cheese (Cheddar or colby); or in one egg
- 8 grams of protein in 1 cup of low-fat milk, 1 cup of beans, 2 tablespoons of peanut butter, 4 ounces of tofu, or ³⁄₄ cup of yogurt
- 2 grams of protein in 1 cup of cooked carrots or green beans
- 3 grams of protein per serving for most starchy foods, such as a slice of bread, ¹⁄₄ cup of cooked pasta, or one small potato

Here are some other ways to make sure you're safely getting the high-quality protein you need.

REAL-LIFE SCENARIO
She Lost Weight but Stayed Flabby

When Margot turned 30, she promised herself that she would go on a diet-and-exercise program to take off the extra 15 pounds that she had put on since college. Ten years and another 20 pounds later, she got around to keeping her promise—or the diet half of it, anyway. She decided that she didn't need the exercise half after reading somewhere that working out is not an efficient way to lose weight. Her diet has worked. She has lost 27 of her extra 35 pounds. But she still isn't happy. Her body is much thinner but no less flabby and saggy. She can wear smaller-size clothes, but they don't look very good on her. Margot has lost hope. It seems that there is no way for her to look good, no matter what she weighs. Or is there?

There sure is. Margot went with half the recipe and wound up with half-baked results. She found out the hard way that looking thinner is not the same thing as looking (and feeling) good. But she can do something about that right now by making exercise a part of her life.

True, a reduced-calorie diet will take off the pounds faster than aerobic exercise alone will. But Margot is in danger of putting those pounds back on. She needs to take advantage of aerobic exercise's fat-burning prowess so she can maintain her weight loss with healthy eating, rather than with a diet that makes her feel deprived.

Keep it coming. Add some protein to most meals and snacks, Wolper says. "When you eat protein with carbohydrates, it helps to stabilize both blood glucose (sugar) levels and insulin levels. Lower insulin levels mean your body is less likely to store glucose as fat." Protein is also satisfying and wards off hunger longer than meals that contain only carbohydrates.

Make a shake. If you're not getting enough protein from your diet or if there are some meals when you want some protein but don't have time to fix something, protein powders are an option, Whittle says. You can find them in your local

More important, Margot needs to start strength training to overcome her thin-but-flabby dilemma. Strength training will not reverse her hard-won weight loss, but it will improve her shape and put an end to her saga of sagginess. Here's why.

When you lose weight through diet alone, you lose lean body mass as well as fat. What's lean body mass? It's pretty much everything in your body that's not fat, with muscle being the most significant part of it. So you may lose fat, but you lose your source of firmness, too.

When you do resistance training at the same time that you diet, however, you actually build lean body mass as you lose fat. It comes in the form of taut and toned muscles that give your body the lean and sculpted look that you had in mind when you decided to lose weight in the first place.

The good news for Margot is that she doesn't have to put on the pounds and start all over again to get it right. She just needs to add two missing ingredients to her weight-loss recipe—aerobic exercise and strength training.

Expert Consulted
Stella L. Volpe, R.D., Ph.D.
Assistant professor in the department of nutrition
Director of the Center for Nutrition in Sport and Human Performance
University of Massachusetts
Amherst

health food store. The protein in these powders often comes from whey, a protein by-product of cheese production, or from egg whites. You can also get soy protein powders. Because soybeans are a good source of protein and calcium, having a soy protein shake may be one easy way to build strong bones and lower the risk of fractures. You can mix any of these powders with water or juice to make low-fat, protein-rich shakes. People with a history of kidney problems or other medical conditions may not need the additional protein in their diets and should consult their doctors or dietitians, says Whittle.

But be careful not to overdo it. A high-protein diet depletes fluid from the body, making dehydration a real risk, Clark says. "That's why people who go on high-protein diets initially lose a lot of water weight."

"Because it is stored solely as fat, excess protein will also eventually lead to weight gain," Wolper adds.

Forgo the aminos. In addition to protein powders, you can find supplements of individual amino acids in health food stores and bodybuilding gyms. Amino acids are the smaller parts that are strung together to make proteins. Bodybuilders often take the supplements to build muscle.

The thinking behind supplements of individual amino acids is that getting more of certain amino acids will somehow help to preserve or increase muscle mass. But much more research needs to be done before any of these substances can be recommended.

"There are many unanswered questions about these substances," Wolper says. If they were drugs, they wouldn't even be on the market. "For now, it's best to simply get adequate protein through foods in your diet.

Fuel Up with Carbs

It's true that carbohydrates—starch and sugar—break down quickly to provide your body with energy. Energy bars, sports drinks, even the sugar-laden gel packets that runners can suck down without stopping . . . all operate on the premise that sugar should be handy and should get into your system fast.

It takes lots of exercise, though—at least 1½ hours of intense activity—to deplete your body

Carb Loading

It's not an excuse to pig out on pasta. It's a technique that some athletes use to get the maximum amount of glycogen (the stored form of sugar) into their muscles for use during an important event. It's supposed to increase stamina.

"This practice may let a well-trained and conditioned athlete go a little longer before she hits the wall, or runs out of gas," says Stacey Whittle, R.D., coauthor of *The Winning Edge of Sports Nutrition* and the nutritionist for the sports nutrition team at Florida Hospital in Orlando. Carbohydrate loading is typically done 1 week before a competition, when athletes reduce their training schedules and rest their muscles to allow them to become saturated with a high-carbohydrate diet.

But do *you* need to carb load? Not unless you're running a marathon or participating in some other all-out event that goes for more than 1½ hours. If you're only doing an hour or so of intense exercise, you can get all the energy you need from well-timed snacks that include carbohydrates, Whittle says. If you haven't eaten in more than 2 to 3 hours, have a snack that includes carbohydrates 30 minutes to 1 hour before your workout. Half a bagel or a piece of toast and some peanut butter or cheese, yogurt with fruit, or a bowl of cereal will all suffice.

of glucose (sugar) and glycogen, the stored form of glucose. You know when that happens. It's called hitting the wall, and it makes your muscles feel like they've turned into lead. Getting some sugar and fluid into you can make all the difference in the world when that happens, says Clark.

Even if you don't work out long enough to hit the wall, exercising first thing in the morning, without having eaten first, or late in the day, long after lunch, can leave your blood sugar low enough to have your tail dragging. Your workout is no fun.

If you consistently eat a diet that's too low in carbohydrates and continue to work out, after a few days, your muscle glycogen stores can fall to less than 50 percent of normal. Such low levels can contribute to feelings of tiredness, soreness, and fatigue. "It's always worth paying attention to your diet to see what could be going on if you feel tired," Whittle says.

Obviously, carbohydrates are important to your body's welfare. Here are some tips that will start you on your way to getting the carbs you need.

Choose calories wisely. You should get about 60 percent of your calories from carbohydrates. Most of that should be from complex carbohydrates—starch such as wheat, potatoes, and pasta. Fruits and vegetables also provide complex carbohydrates. And if you stick with whole-grain starches such as wholewheat bread, oatmeal, brown rice, and the like, you'll be doing yourself an additional favor by getting more fiber, which slows digestion and helps you feel fuller, Whittle says.

Go low-sugar. Keep your calorie intake from sugar down to about 10 percent. Sugar offers nothing in the way of nutrients. If you're on a 1,500-calorie diet, that comes to 150 calories a day from sugar, or about 38 grams. You can find sugar content, listed in grams, on the labels of the foods you eat. One energy bar contains 16 grams of sugar, for example, and one serving (8 ounces) of a sports drink, 14 grams.

Figure in Fat

Once you've gotten your protein and carbohydrate needs met, the rest of your calories—the remaining 15 to 20 percent—can come from fat, says Whittle.

Fat is an important part of any diet. We all need some fat, especially to produce hormones, regulate metabolism, and form the structures of cell membranes. And it provides a source of energy for exercise and activity.

Fat is also very satisfying and wards off hunger for a long time, so you don't want to avoid it entirely, Whittle says. "It's interesting to see how a moderate-to-low fat intake affects a person's weight and hunger. The days of no-fat diets are over—they just don't work. Fat is not going to make you fat unless you are consuming more calories than you need."

The kind of fat you eat can make a big difference in your health. Go easy on saturated fats by choosing low-fat cheeses and dairy products and lean cuts of meat, Whittle recommends. Also go easy on hydrogenated fats, which are fats that have been converted into an even more saturated form, by avoiding the products that often contain them, such as margarine and processed baked goods. Instead, get your fat from fish like salmon, mackerel, sardines, herring, and tuna, which offer heart-healthy omega-6 and -3 fatty acids. And consider adding 1 tablespoon of ground flaxseed or 1 teaspoon of flaxseed oil to your daily diet since more than half its fat is composed of omega-3 fatty acids and may help with hormonal balance during menopause. "I also like to recommend nuts and seeds—natural peanut butter or sunflowers," Whittle says. "These foods stay with you longer and provide some protein. They tend to help keep blood sugar normal, too. You need to eat them moderately since too much of a good thing can be fattening."

Get Your Eight-a-Day

You need water to live. You also need it to perform well. Even mild dehydration—as little as a 1 percent loss in body weight—can hurt your performance by causing dizziness, headache, and slower-than-normal reaction times. Exercise can actually disrupt your normal

WOMEN ASK WHY

Why can't I just eat some energy bars and forget about my diet?

No doubt about it, energy bars are convenient and a good thing to have on hand when you're out on a long bike ride or hike. And they can make a decent afternoon snack. But don't make the mistake that many women do of trying to live on them or of substituting them for real meals. One a day as a 200-calorie snack is okay, as long as you're not overeating.

Read the fine print on the label before you decide on a bar. Not all energy bars are created equal. Some are quite nutritious. Clif bars, for example, contain fiber, protein, vitamins, and minerals, and have no hydrogenated fat. And high-protein bars won't give you a spike in blood sugar the way a bar that contains lots of refined sugar would. Many bars, however, are made mostly from sugar, and some also contain palm oil or hydrogenated vegetable oil—both fats that you should avoid.

Expert Consulted
Stacey Whittle, R.D.
Coauthor of The Winning Edge of Sports Nutrition
Nutritionist for the sports nutrition team at Florida Hospital in Orlando

WHAT'S UP WITH THIS?

"Fat Burner" Drinks

You may see them at health foods stores or even at your gym. They're "fat burner" or "thermogenic" or "metabolic" products. But do they really work? And just what's in them?

Most contain a number of ingredients. Some, called E-C-A stacks, contain a patented mix of ephedrine and caffeine (both stimulants) and aspirin. These products work by revving up cells to waste energy as excess heat instead of storing it as fat, explains Carla Wolper, R.D., a nutritionist at the Obesity Research Center at St. Luke's–Roosevelt Hospital Center in New York City. "Ephedrine and caffeine act synergistically to increase metabolism and decrease appetite, and the small amount of aspirin in the capsules blocks a feedback mechanism in cells that would otherwise slow down the increase," Wolper says.

The E-C-A combination has been proven to "support modest, sustained weight loss even without prescribed calorie restriction," in the words of one research group. In one study, people taking an E-C-A stack lost an average of about 11½ pounds in 5 months, compared to a no-intervention group, who each gained less than 1 pound. And several studies have found that the E-C-A stack targets body fat while preserving muscle.

The downside? These products have the potential to cause irregular heartbeat, headaches, anxiety, insomnia, and jitteriness. "These side effects may be worse in the first week or so, but then, as your body adapts, they may disappear," Wolper says. Still, people with high blood pressure, heart disease, or other medical conditions, including pregnancy, are advised not to use these products. "Talk with your doctor first, get a good physical, make sure you have no underlying heart disease, and have your blood pressure monitored," Wolper adds. "Then, if she gives you the okay, follow the label directions."

thirst mechanism, so you can become dehydrated without feeling thirsty, says Susan Kleiner, R.D., Ph.D., a private nutrition consultant to athletes in the Seattle area and a member of the American Dietetics Association's Sports and Cardiovascular Nutritionists group.

Sports drinks do offer performance advantages over juice or water. Properly formulated sports drinks can speed water into the body more quickly than drinking water alone, Dr. Kleiner says. The key element is the carbohydrate solution, which should range from 6 to 8 percent. "This concentration appears to activate a glucose pump in the intestines that pumps both water and carbohydrates into the bloodstream at a faster rate than plain water is absorbed," Dr. Kleiner says. A 6 to 8 percent solution also has been shown to prolong exercise time, particularly for aerobic activities that last longer than 60 minutes. Sports drinks should contain a mixture of fructose (fruit sugar), which gives an initial burst of energy, and glucose polymers, often called maltodextrin on product labels, Dr. Kleiner says.

However, if weight loss, not performance, is your main goal, you may not want to consume sports drinks while you exercise, says Whittle. "Instead of burning the fat on your body, you are using carbohydrates from the sports drink as some of your fuel," she explains. You will burn more fat if you stick with water as your fluid. Plan on drinking about ½ to ¾ cup of fluid every 15 minutes during a workout. After your activity, weigh yourself and drink 2 cups of water for every pound of weight you lost during the workout.

If plain old H_2O bores you, add an orange or

lemon herbal tea bag to your chilled water bottle.

The Vitals on Vitamins

If you are on a weight-loss diet, many nutritionists recommend that you take a multivitamin-and-mineral pill, "just to cover your bases," says Dr. Kleiner. Women tend to come up short on a number of nutrients—iron, calcium, folic acid, B$_6$—and even more so when they're trying to cut back on calories. Vitamins and minerals are essential for every body function, including building muscles and burning fat. Deficiencies of vitamins, especially some of the B vitamins, can cause a reduction in physical performance. However, getting more of these vitamins than you need isn't going to give you extra energy.

Look for a multivitamin/mineral that offers 100 percent or close to 100 percent of the Daily Value of all of the 13 vitamins and 15 minerals that are considered essential for human health, Dr. Kleiner recommends.

"Some vitamins and minerals are advertised as being especially important for muscle-building and weight loss, but really, they're just a waste of time and money," Dr. Kleiner says. These include chromium and vanadium. While it's important to get adequate amounts of these trace minerals, there is no need for the high amounts found in some supplements.

However, there is one vitamin you should get more of: vitamin E, which appears to minimize oxygen-related damage that occurs to muscles

during exercise and to reduce muscle soreness in older women. Dr. Kleiner recommends you take 100 to 400 international units of vitamin E a day. If your multivitamin supplement doesn't contain E, you'll have to take a separate vitamin pill. Talk to your doctor if you plan on taking more than 200 international units of vitamin E daily.

Toning and the "Older" Woman

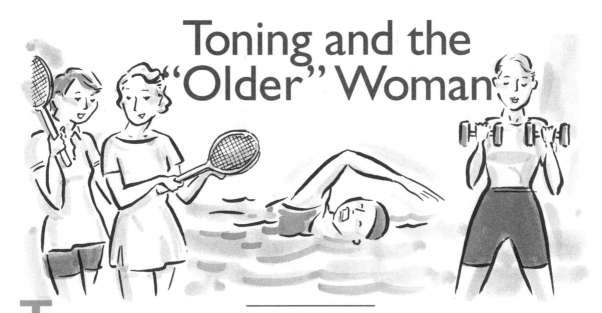

here's only one important difference between a rocking chair and the electric chair: one of them, you have to plug in.

Sit in either for too long, and the result can be the same.

To remain healthy as you get older, you have to stay active and strong, and that doesn't happen when you're constantly sitting in a rocking chair and knitting. It's use it or lose it, where muscles are concerned.

"Most women lose about ⅓ to ½ pound of muscle a year after age 35. By the time they're 80, some can't perform even routine tasks, like getting up out of a chair or climbing stairs," says Miriam Nelson, Ph.D., director of the Center for Physical Fitness at Tufts University School of Nutrition Science and Policy in Boston and author of *Strong Women Stay Young* and *Strong Women Stay Slim*.

Part of this loss of strength is from aging, "but it's also from inactivity, and *that* you can do something about," Dr. Nelson says. "Research shows that people who strength train seem to preserve their youthful body compositions very well."

Dr. Nelson's own studies show that women in their fifties and sixties who do high-intensity strength training can develop strength scores more typical of women in their late thirties or early forties. "We have seen an increase in muscle mass in people even in their nineties," she says. "I'm not saying we are going to make a 90-year-old look like a 20-year-old, but we can see the body shape change to take on a more youthful appearance."

Boning Up on Exercise

What's true for muscle is also true for bones, Dr. Nelson says. Use 'em or lose 'em.

Unless women take replacement hormones, we can lose up to 20 percent of bone mass in the first 5 to 7 years after menopause, followed by a continuous, slower loss. But exercise that stresses the bone, such as high-intensity strength training, can change that. It can actually preserve bone mass; and in some cases, it even leads to a slight increase, says Dr. Nelson.

"Even that slight increase, or just maintaining bone mass, is important," Dr. Nelson says. "The alternative is allowing your bones to become so brittle and weak over time that you can begin to have fractures."

So no matter what your age, today is the day to start exercising. Even women who already have osteoporosis can strength train, as long as they start out very slowly. While they probably won't regain enough bone mass to stop potential fractures, they can regain muscle strength, which will help them maintain balance and prevent falls, Dr. Nelson says. But she cautions, "Women who have osteoporosis need to work with their doctors to develop a total program, which includes exercise, nutritional support, and, perhaps, drugs."

Make the Most of Your Efforts

Here's what you need to know to make the most of your exercise regimen—and stick with it.

Weight for it. If you want to increase muscle strength and bone density, you have to use weights heavy enough to "max out" at 8 to 10 reps, Dr. Nelson says. "When you do lots of repetitions with lighter weights, you build endurance, not strength. That's fine, except aerobic exercise does this far more effi-

WOMAN TO WOMAN
She's Fit at 56

Lois Crawford, a registered dietitian from Mount Pleasant, Texas, waited until her child-rearing years were complete before she started a regular exercise program. And she was in her fifties when she added strength training to her workout schedule. Now 56, Lois has discovered all of the good things that working with weights offers women of any age, plus some other benefits that younger exercisers may not have considered.

I didn't really make any conscious effort to get into strength training. But 3 years ago, when I enrolled in a body-conditioning class at the local community college, it turned out that weight training was part of the program. So there I was, at age 53, starting to lift weights. I've certainly never regretted it.

For one thing, I like the exercising itself—both the weights and my aerobic work. I like to do it at home alone and with a group. Each has its advantages. At home, I exercise on my own schedule in my climate-controlled living room. With the group, there's camaraderie and fun.

And of course, I love the results, starting with my appearance. You'd have a hard time finding any flab on me. I'm not saying that I'm petite, but not much jiggles.

Another thing is posture. I was a frequent sloucher before, but now I find that I've lost that round-shouldered look. That's a sure way to look younger!

Aside from appearance, weight training has done some other things for me. For one, it has improved my balance. I'm even more sure on my feet when I'm getting in and out of a boat.

My flexibility has also improved. When I need to back up in my car, for example, turning around in my seat to see behind me is much easier.

Maybe the most welcome benefit of all at my age is the energy I feel. The combination of aerobic exercise and strength training has helped me do things that lots of women in their twenties could only dream of. For example, I just got back from finishing a 7-day, 500-mile bike tour of Texas.

All in all, I'd describe myself as a compact, energetic, and sunny-dispositioned 56-year-old; and my positive self-image comes from exercise.

"You should progress slowly, increasing your weight about 10 percent every 2 to 3 weeks at first," she says. Make sure that you're able to lift the weight at least 10 times before moving on to the next weight level. "Your bones will get stronger, just as your muscles do, but they need more time to develop."

Get help. If you're working out at a gym and using exercise machines for the first time, find someone who can instruct you at your level, says Dr. Rikli. "There's only one thing worst than no exercise at all, and that's too much, where you damage a joint. Someone who knows how to instruct older people can make sure they start out at a safe level."

Warm up and cool down. Older bodies take time to get in the mood for exercise, get more blood flowing into muscles, and limber up, Dr. Nelson says. Conversely, they also need more time to slow heart rate and cool off after a workout, she adds. "Even just standing and then sitting down in a chair 8 to 12 times is a good warmup. So is going up a couple of flights of stairs. It takes about 5 minutes to really get the blood flowing." Alternately, you can do one set of each exercise without any weights to get your muscles warmed up and blood flowing.

A proper warmup helps reduce your risk for injuries because it helps your muscles to work at their optimum level. And, along with cooldown, it's mandatory if you have heart disease, says

ciently." Lifting poundage that's too easy for you also means you miss out on bone benefits. Studies indicate that only women who do high-intensity lifting protect or boost their bone density.

Start slowly. Even if you can only lift 2 pounds when you start out, that's fine, says Roberta Rikli, Ph.D., chairperson of the department of kinesiology and health promotion at California State University in Fullerton.

Carol Garber, Ph.D., clinical exercise physiologist and director of the Human Performance Laboratory at Memorial Hospital of Rhode Island in Pawtucket.

"You can get light-headed or have chest pains from angina if you start or stop too quickly," Dr. Garber says. And some medications for high blood pressure or heart disease make your body warm up and cool down more slowly than normal, she adds. A 5 to 10 minute warmup is adequate for most people, on or off medication. However, if you're feeling particularly stiff or sluggish, give yourself a few more minutes.

Don't be a heartbreaker. If you're afraid to exercise because you have heart disease, your doctor can write you a prescription for cardiac rehabilitation, which allows you to learn to exercise in a safe, monitored environment, Dr. Garber says. The best place for such exercise is in a cardiac rehabilitation program in a hospital or other health facility, where medical personnel can monitor you.

Start big. After your warmup, work the large muscles of your trunk and legs first. You want to target these big, important muscles while you have maximum energy. Hitting them first also helps your smaller muscle groups prepare for the work to come, Dr. Nelson says.

Do squats. "They're great because they target a lot of muscles," Dr. Nelson says. Some women may need to begin by squatting down only 1 to 2 inches to begin with, doing modi-

---

WHAT'S UP WITH THIS?
Facial Exercises (and Why They Don't Work)

"Facercises." "Facemetrics." "Five-Minute Facelift." The creators of facial exercise programs say their regimens can erase years and signs of stress in just minutes a day. "You exercise your body. Why not your face?" asks one ad for Facial Magic, a videotape that promises you'll look 10 to 15 years younger once you begin its program. Good question.

Unfortunately, no facial exercise program is scientifically proven to reduce wrinkles, says Beverly Fischer, M.D., a surgeon in Timonium, Maryland, and clinical instructor in the department of plastic surgery at Johns Hopkins Hospital in Baltimore. "Your face develops wrinkles from sun exposure, aging, and the pull of gravity, not from weak muscles," she says. "The underlying musculature can play a small role in exaggerating wrinkles, but these muscles are so small that you can't really build them up enough to reduce facial lines."

Facial exercises can be helpful, however, in helping people to recover after a bout of Bell's palsy, which paralyzes facial muscles, or after a stroke that affects the face.

---

fied squats from a chair. "Just getting up and down from a chair is a good way to start," she says.

Rest up. Give your muscles 48 hours between sessions. Strength training two or three times a week is great for women of all ages, Dr. Nelson says. "Even older women can recover within 48 hours," she says. If you don't recover within this period of time, you are doing too much during your sessions. You'll know that you overdid it if you are still very stiff and it's painful to move your muscles through their full range of motion.

Use free weights and machines. Both have advantages and disadvantages, Dr. Rikli says. Weight machines make you maintain proper form and help prevent injuries if you lose control of the weight. Free weights, on the other hand, require additional coordination, balance, and proper body alignment—they take more work, but you always have complete control of the movements. They're also inexpensive, they don't take up much storage space, and they're portable.

Use real weights, not soup cans. Soup cans aren't heavy enough for most women to develop strength, Dr. Nelson says. And don't use milk jugs filled with sand or water, either, she cautions. The jugs put your wrists in an awkward position that can cause damage over time.

Invest in some decent workout togs. A couple of good sports bras can prevent painful back and shoulder problems; and stretchy, form-fitting fabrics such as spandex, which exert pressure on muscles, can increase your output and endurance, according to a study done at Pennsylvania State University in University Park.

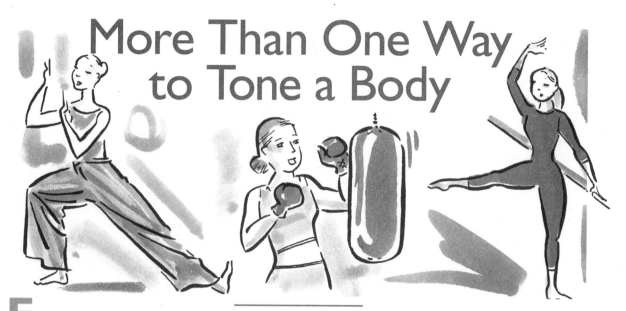

More Than One Way to Tone a Body

For some of us, lifting weights becomes a joy—an expression of our physical and emotional strength, a boost to our body images, a spirit-cleansing source of stress relief.

Then there are the rest of us, who know (or suspect) that hefting barbells and dumbbells, or using weight machines, would drive us batty if that were our only exercise.

But if you think that pumping iron is the only way to get a fitter, firmer body, think again. "You don't have to lift weights to get the benefits of resistance training," says Amanda L. Johnson, a certified personal trainer in Chicago. "There are other types of resistance training that provide similar physiological benefits and that you may find more enjoyable."

So if you've decided that you prefer a low-iron workout regimen, no problem. There are plenty of other muscle-firming workouts to try, from the slow, gentle rhythms of Pilates to the frenetic pace of some marital-arts-style workouts, such as cardio kickboxing.

Most of the activities below use your own body weight as resistance. They can be used as a primary strength-training program or, in some cases, as a supplement to it. One of them is bound to appeal to you, whether you're new to exercise or a habitual exerciser looking for a fun, new way to stay strong.

Before participating in any of the activities mentioned below, discuss with the instructor any health conditions that you may have, says Geralyn Coopersmith, exercise physiologist, certified strength-conditioning specialist, and certified personal trainer at The Trainer's Place in New York City. These include pregnancy, high blood pressure, glaucoma, and back problems. Once your teacher knows your limitations, she can modify difficult poses and movements or steer you away from those that are unsafe for you.

Step Up to the Barre

If your inner child wears a tutu and a tiara, consider supplementing your resistance training with ballet classes. You may not develop a ballerina's chiseled body, but you will get toning benefits and improve your flexibility, a vital component of a good fitness program, says

Christine Spizzo, an instructor of dance education at New York University in New York City, who has danced with Mikhail Baryshnikov and Rudolf Nureyev and currently performs in *The Phantom of the Opera* on Broadway.

Adult beginners' ballet classes are offered everywhere. Just look in the Yellow Pages under "Dancing Instruction."

Most classes are 90-minutes long, including warmup and cooldown time. Wear fitted clothing that allows you to move freely, yet still allows you to see the shape of your body. Spizzo suggests stretchy cotton or cotton-blend warmup pants—not sweats—over a snapless leotard. (You don't want to unsnap with one leg over the barre.) You'll also need ballet slippers with leather bottoms to give your feet traction while still allowing them to turn and slide.

The Power of the Sword

You won't swing from chandeliers, brandishing a saber like in the old Errol Flynn movies. But fencing will give you an intense workout that will build muscle without bulk, says Gary Guerriero, physical therapist, certified athletic trainer, co-owner of the U.S. Athletic Training Center in New York City, and coauthor of *Get a Gold Medal Butt.*

Fencing is a great lower-body workout, says Guerriero. Its quick, explosive motions— lunges, advances, and retreats—work the hips, legs, and butt. And while it requires mental

REAL-LIFE SCENARIO
She'd Rather Be Dancing

Jennifer hates to exercise. She'd rather sit around waiting for light bulbs to burn out than join her husband when he pounds weights in the home gym that he bought and set up in the basement. On the other hand, she loves to dance. She doesn't think about it, she just does it, whether she's doing movements from her childhood ballet class or a funky disco step. Whenever there's music, she's up and moving—and in her home, there is *always* music. Now, she wants to take swing-dancing lessons, but her husband, who thinks she's in terrible shape because she never exercises, will agree to go only if she agrees to start working out regularly with him. He says he's concerned for her health and pesters her endlessly. Meanwhile, the registration deadline for the dance class is looming. Should she give in? Maybe her husband is right and she does need to join him in the "dungeon," as she calls it.

Jennifer's husband should stop nagging. Those pliés and the Hustle absolutely count as exercise. If she's dancing at a high intensity for 5 to 10 minutes several times a day (for a total of 20 minutes or more), she's strengthening her cardiovascular system, a vital component of any fitness program, and she's getting a mini muscle-endurance workout, using her body weight as resistance. She's also increasing her flexibility.

But while Jennifer's legs are probably in fabulous shape, chances are, her upper body isn't. So even if she "hates" to exercise, Jennifer should join her man in the dungeon, or find another activity that improves muscle tone, such as Pilates or power yoga. She would gain the benefits of cross-training,

discipline, much like ballet or the martial arts, it's also a great stress reliever. "You get to strike things, but no one gets hurt," says Guerriero.

Beginners typically fence for 20 to 30 minutes, three times a week, and eventually work

which is simply a fancy term for varying your exercise programs.

Cross-training—combining calisthenics with cycling, say, or kickboxing with swimming—is the best way to build peak strength, flexibility, and endurance. When you cross-train, you improve muscle fitness, which will give you more endurance and make you less prone to injury. In Jennifer's case, her dancing takes care of her flexibility and endurance. Resistance training would build muscle, particularly in her upper body.

To be in peak form, Jennifer should do some form of resistance training two or three times a week, for a minimum of 15 to 30 minutes at a time. She can make her time in the dungeon more bearable by listening to her favorite swing music during workouts and telling herself that she's in training for her swing-dancing lessons. This style of dance is strenuous, so she'll need that upper-body strength.

But Jennifer's husband isn't completely off the hook. He should join his wife on the dance floor. He'd benefit as much from dancing as Jennifer would from weight training. Dancing just 20 minutes per day, 3 to 5 days a week, would increase his cardiovascular health and flexibility, which would help prevent weight-training injuries and give him a heart-healthy workout as well.

Expert Consulted
Geralyn Coopersmith
Exercise physiologist, certified strength-conditioning specialist, and certified personal trainer
The Trainer's Place
New York City

their way up to an hour, says Guerriero. Show up for class in sweats and sneakers; the fencing school will provide the mask, sword (called a foil), and other equipment. If you decide to stay with the sport, some mail-order companies offer starter packages that include a mask, jacket, glove, and foil. A basic set costs from $100 to $200.

To find a fencing class in your area, call the local YWCA/YMCA or check the Yellow Pages under "Fencing." Or contact area universities; many have fencing teams and may offer instruction as well, says Guerriero. You can also write to the U.S. Fencing Association, One Olympic Plaza, Colorado Springs, CO 80909, to request a welcome packet, which includes a state-by-state listing of fencing instructors.

Ready to Get Firm? Get Inline

Remember your 8-, 9-, or 10-year-old self who glided giddily around the neighborhood on her roller skates? Inline skating can give you back that feeling—and firm your butt in the bargain. It's a full-body workout that strengthens the muscles of your legs, hips, buttocks, abdomen, chest, upper back, shoulders, and arms.

For maximum benefit, skate for an hour three times a week, recommends Elizabeth Yastrzemski, an inline-skating instructor in Southhampton, New York, who is certified by the International Inline Skating Association (IISA) in Wilmington, North Carolina. You really must skate, as opposed to glide. "Skate against the wind," says Yastrzemski. "Once you know what you're doing, you can skate uphill, which will really work your hips and butt."

Take a lesson or two from a certified instructor before you go off on your own, recommends Yastrzemski. Skate shops or sporting goods stores are good places to find them. Or write to IISA's Instructor Certification Program at 201 North Front Street #306, Wilmington, NC 28401.

Because new, good-quality skates can cost from $150 to $200, ask your instructor if you can rent skates while you take lessons. Whether or not you choose to take lessons, always wear a helmet, protective wrist guards, and elbow and knee pads. And if you're a beginner, skate on paved pathways in the park, not on the road.

Fitness, Asian Style

Tae Bo is one hybrid form of boxing and martial arts, also referred to as kickboxing, cardio kickboxing, or cardio boxing. Whatever you call it, a martial-arts-style aerobics class is "a fantastic full-body workout that firms and tones muscles as it strengthens your cardiovascular system," says Johnson.

While cardio kickboxing will tone your entire body, it's a particularly effective upper-body workout, says Johnson. Throwing jabs, cross jabs, and hooks will give you nicely shaped arms and shoulders, while the leg work—front snap kicks and roundhouse kicks—will tone your hips, thighs, and buttocks.

The typical cardio-kickboxing class is structured much like a aerobics class, says Johnson. After a brief warmup, you swing

---

HOME, SWEET GYM

Can't afford to join a gym? No problem. If you have at least 5 square feet of space, you can set up your own personal "health club" for less than $100, says Geralyn Coopersmith, exercise physiologist, certified strength-conditioning specialist, and certified personal trainer at The Trainer's Place in New York City. Here's what you need to build your health-club-for-one.

A step bench: $0 to $40. Used in step aerobics, these sturdy plastic benches can be found in the sporting goods section of many large department stores such as Kmart or Wal-Mart. "You can do a total-body workout on a bench with just some free weights," says Coopersmith. Use it for upper-body work such as dumbbell flies, pullovers, chest presses, and bent rows, and for leg work such as one-legged squats and step-ups.

To save money, use a sturdy piano bench or a coffee table without a glass top. If you go this route, make sure your bench supports your weight and doesn't wobble.

An assortment of dumbbells: about $25. To start, buy one pair each of 3-, 5-, and 7-pound dumbbells. Purchase solid-metal dumbbells (available at sporting goods stores and department stores, or by mail order) for more dollar value, advises Coopersmith. They're significantly cheaper than the chrome variety. As you progress in your program, purchase 15- and 20-pound dumbbells.

An exercise mat: $10 and up. You'll need it for pelvic tilts, crunches, and other floor exercises. You should look

---

into the routine, which consists of punching and kicking techniques performed both separately and in combination and usually to music.

Most health clubs offer martial-arts-style workouts, as may the YWCA or YMCA, says Johnson. Try a martial-arts academy, too—some now offer cardio-kickboxing classes as well as their traditional programs. Wear basic workout

for a mat with 1-inch-thick polyethylene foam for durability. Also, it shouldn't be either too firm or too squishy.

As you progress in your program, consider purchasing the items below, available at department or sporting goods stores or through mail-order health-and-fitness catalogs.

Resistance bands: $10 to $15. These oversized rubber bands are an inexpensive way to add variety to your workout. You work your upper and lower body by stretching them in various directions. (Instructions are included.) They're usually sold in sets of three or four, and each band has a different level of resistance. As one band becomes too easy, you progress to the next.

A physio ball: $12 and up. "You can do tons of exercises with physio balls, including abdominal, leg, and lower-back work," says Coopersmith. "I sometimes give my clients entire workouts on them." Physio balls are sized in centimeters, and the size that you should buy depends on your height. If you're 5 feet 1 inch to 5 feet 6 inches, for example, you'd need a ball that's 55 centimeters wide. When you sit on it, your knees should be at a 90-degree angle. Ball pumps cost $8.50 and up.

A medicine ball: $20 and up. Unlike physio balls, medicine balls are weighted, making them ideal for leg squats and lunges, triceps extensions, biceps curls, and more, says Coopersmith. Medicine balls come in varying weights. The more they weigh, the more they cost. To start, buy a 4.4-pound ball, which costs from $25 to $30.

attire, such as shorts, a T-shirt, and aerobics shoes.

In some classes, you spar with a partner. But you won't be socking anyone in the nose. "Many women come up to me before a class and say, 'I'm not a violent person. I don't know if I can do this,'" says Johnson. "But you don't need to think or act violently to take this type of class. The goal is just to get a good workout."

The Dancer's Workout

Practiced by dancers such as Martha Graham and George Balanchine, Pilates (pronounced Puh-LAH-teez) has been discovered by athletes, celebrities, and regular folks who want sleek-yet-powerful muscles.

Despite its growing popularity, many people still harbor misconceptions about this elegant—but physically demanding—mat-and-machine-based workout. "It's not yoga. It's not a stretching technique. It's resistance training, pure and simple," says Alycea Ungaro, a licensed physical therapist and owner of Tribeca Bodyworks in New York City.

Developed by Joseph H. Pilates, a boxer and gymnast who also studied yoga and meditation, Pilates is a system of more than 500 controlled movements that strengthen muscles without adding bulk, using your own body weight as resistance. It's performed either on a floor mat or with special equipment that includes springs, pulleys, chains, and a contraption called the Universal Reformer.

While Pilates strengthens all muscle groups, it focuses on your body's "power center"—the muscles of your abdomen, buttocks, and lower back, says Ungaro. In fact, Pilates is ideal for people with back problems, because it's a low-impact workout that doesn't stress joints or ligaments.

You'll get the best results if you do Pilates for 1 hour three times a week, says Ungaro. You can do the floor work at home, but most people also attend outside classes to use the equipment.

MAKE A (LOVE) MUSCLE

Yes, muscle tone makes us look better in bathing suits. But it also comes in mighty handy when we make love.

Specifically, we're talking about the pubococcygeal (PC) muscles which run from the public bone to the tailbone. "The PC are used during intercourse and contract during orgasm," says Elizabeth Lee Vliet, M.D., founder and medical director of HER Place: Health Enhancement and Renewal for Women in Tucson, Arizona, and in Dallas/Fort Worth. According to some experts, giving your PC a regular workout can lead to stronger, more intense orgasms.

Here's how to whip those love muscles into shape.

Get to know them. To find your PC muscles, sit on the toilet and stop and start your flow of urine, says Dr. Vliet.

Put on the squeeze. Contract the PC hard for 1 second, then release, says Dr. Vliet. Repeat 15 to 20 times. Do two sets of regular, short squeezes—called Kegels—twice a day. Gradually work up to two sets of 75 per day.

Continue to train. When you can do 150 short squeezes a day, add a series of long Kegel squeezes, says Dr. Vliet. Simply perform the regular Kegel, but hold the contraction for a count of three. Relax your PC between contractions. Start with two sets of 20 long Kegels and work up to 75. (You'll then be doing 300 a day—150 long squeezes, 150 short.)

At this point, you'll be ready to do "pushouts." After relaxing your PC, push down and out *gently*—don't bear down, says Dr. Vliet.

Maintain your muscle. Combine long and short Kegels with pushouts. In 2 months, your PC muscles should be as well-toned as your biceps. "To keep it that way, do 150 repetitions several times a week," says Dr. Vliet.

and taught the technique for many years and is certified to teach Pilates. To find a certified instructor in your area, write to The Pilates Studio, 890 Broadway, Sixth Floor, New York, NY 10003.

Meditation with Muscle

You won't find practitioners of power yoga in the lotus position, at least not until the end of their workout. Unlike some other forms of yoga, they're busy sweating and getting *strong* before they get to this final posture.

Drawn from a branch of classic yoga called astanga, power yoga is a series of intense yoga movements. But there's no resting time between poses, which is why it's such rigorous exercise.

Despite its intensity, power yoga is an all-ages workout. "Most of the women I teach are in their mid-twenties to their mid-fifties, and one of my students is 73," says Christina Allen, owner of Astanga Yoga Center East in San Marcos, California, who has been practicing astanga yoga for 10 years and teaching for 4.

Many health clubs offer classes in power yoga, and many instructors teach out of their homes. Wear loose clothing and no socks. Classes typically run about 1 hour to 1 hour and 15 minutes, and you should attend twice a week for maximum benefit. Class size varies; a class offered by a health club may have 30 students, while a session

You'll start out with one-on-one instruction and progress to small groups.

Many health clubs offer Pilates-style workouts. Make sure your instructor has studied

taught by a private instructor may have as few as 3. But no matter how big the group, you'll get individual attention. The instructor walks around the room to adjust everyone's pose.

A Real Swingin' Workout

A blend of high-energy moves and old-fashioned charm, swing dancing evolved from the lindy in the 1930s and flowered in the Big Band era of the 1940s. It has made a comeback, and, as many people have discovered, it's a great workout.

Dancing two or three times a week will firm the muscles in your legs, hips, buttocks, arms, back, and shoulders, says Johnson. It will also increase your muscular endurance.

Just ask Annie Hirsch of Corona del Mar, California, who has been swing dancing for 50 years. "I'm 70 years old, and I can still dance for hours because dancing gives you sustained endurance," says the champion-level swing-dance-competition coordinator and judge.

Many universities offer swing-dancing classes, as do adult-education classes and the YWCA/YMCA. To find dances in your area, check your newspaper's weekend section. Most dances include an hour-long beginners' lesson, followed by dancing to music provided by a disc jockey or band.

WHAT'S UP WITH THIS?
Isometrics

Remember that breast-building exercise that you used to do when you were 13, in which you pushed your palms together in front of your chest as hard as you could umpteen times a day? That's one example of an isometric exercise. In isometrics, you either push against an immovable object, such as a wall, or simply tighten a muscle and hold the contraction.

But while isometric exercise can strengthen muscles, it's no substitute for a regular strength-training program, says Lisa Hoffman, an exercise physiologist; president of Solo Fitness, a personal training company based in New York City; and coauthor of *Better Than Ever: The 4-Week Workout Program for Women over 40*. You need to put stress on a muscle—the principle of "overload"—to increase its size and strength, explains Hoffman. "Isometrics don't work alone as a total body-fitness routine because they don't stress the muscle enough with outside resistance such as a dumbbell or a resistance band."

Also, during an isometric contraction, your muscles don't shorten and lengthen as they do when you lift weights, which requires a full range of motion. So muscle development is limited.

That's not to say that isometrics don't have their place in a fitness program. Many people do them while they're traveling, for example. What's more, isometric exercise can be helpful to people with joint injuries, which is why it's widely used in physical therapy. "Isometric exercise allows you to work the muscle around the affected joint without moving the joint itself," says Hoffman.

Water Fitness with Spirit

When performed against the resistance of water, the graceful movements of tai chi, a traditional Chinese martial art, become a muscle-toning workout. "Water provides about 12 times the resistance of air," says Carol Argo, certified instructor and trainer for the Aquatic Exercise Association (AEA), based in Nokomis, Florida, and owner of The Fitness Company in Palos Verdes, California, who also teaches traditional tai chi. "Water tai chi can help increase your strength and flexibility, especially in your legs, but also in your arms and torso."

Water tai chi is performed upright, in chest-deep water, in a warm-water (about 84 to 88°F)

pool. Most classes last for an hour and consist of cardiovascular exercise, muscle toning, and some sort of relaxation movement. For best results, you should attend two or three times a week, says Argo. Wear your regular bathing suit and aquatic shoes.

To find a water-tai-chi class (or other resistance-exercise classes performed in the water, if tai chi isn't available), start by calling the YWCA/YMCA or area health clubs. Or write to AEA, P.O. Box 1609, Nokomis, FL 34274, to find a certified instructor in your area.

Toning for Keeps

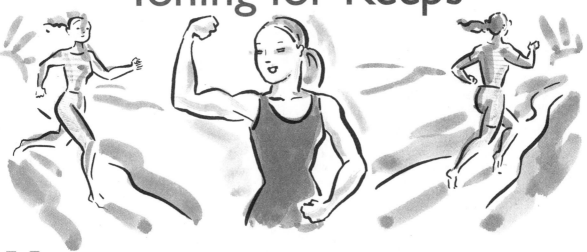

You tell yourself, "It's time to exercise."

Then, a stubborn little voice in the back of your head replies, "Okay . . . only my muscles are stiff, I got up late, I don't have time, and I have a million and one distractions to deal with. Besides, I have as much of a right to be lazy now and then as anybody else does."

"Cut the excuses and just do it," you tell yourself. But will you?

Eventually, whether it's our first workout or our hundredth, we all have this little discussion with ourselves. If we're really committed to exercising, we force ourselves to work out anyway. Afterward, of course, we feel terrific. We've won the struggle.

The problem is that a 40-year-old woman will live, on average, another 40 years. If she intends to work out three times a week for the rest of her life, she'll have to win that struggle roughly 6,240 more times.

Can she?

Of course. Women do it all the time. And not because they possess some mysterious exercise gene that the rest of us don't.

"Women who don't exercise often think that women who do possess some magical quality, or at least more willpower. But it's not true," says Kymberly Williams-Evans, chairperson of the group fitness committee for IDEA, the international organization for health and fitness professionals located in San Diego, and academic advisor for the fitness instruction minor at the University of California in Santa Barbara.

What they do have is knowledge and experience to get them over the rough spots. They've learned how to exercise when they're scraping the bottom of the motivational barrel. How to set challenging yet achievable goals. How to fit exercise into an impossible schedule. How to make working out a form of play. All lessons you'll need to learn if you're going to stick with a fitness program for keeps.

Getting Psyched to Sweat

In the long run, a woman is most likely to stick with a workout program if she clearly knows what she wants to get out of it: better health, stress relief, or just a great body. But

No woman "hates" to exercise. What she hates are her preconceived notions about exercise—that it's painful and inconvenient, that she doesn't do it correctly, that it's a chore rather than an activity that can be both fun and beneficial to her physical and emotional well-being.

When women associate exercise with physical pain, it's often because they lifted more weight than they should have or did too many repetitions during their first visits to the gym. When they couldn't move the next day, they blamed the exercise itself, rather than an overambitious workout.

Other women think they dislike exercise because they feel foolish doing it. They think that it requires physical skill or feel pressured to exercise flawlessly, much in the way they feel pressured to be perfect mothers or perfect workers. But doing an arm curl or leg extension doesn't require any unique skills whatsoever.

Women may also hate working out because they believe it should be unpleasant or boring—that if it feels good, it can't possibly have any serious benefits. But, as many women who have "hated" exercise have learned, exercise comes in many different forms. You just have to find the form that works for you, whether it's Pilates or power yoga, kickboxing or bicycling in the park.

If you "hate" to exercise, challenge your assumptions about it. Then try to reframe your idea of exercise in a positive light. Think of it as a gift from you to yourself, as a time-out from the hustle and bustle of your daily life.

Remember, too, that it takes some time to make exercise a habit—at least 6 weeks. If you can stick to an exercise program for this long, you may find that, far from "hating" exercise, you actually look forward to your workouts.

Expert Consulted
Judith Young, Ph.D.
Executive director, National Association for
*   Sport and Physical Education*
Reston, Virginia

along the road, she may also come to love the way it feels to have toned, strong, responsive muscles, and that in itself may motivate her.

"If you stay with your program long enough, you discover the joy of having a body that will do what you want it to do," says LaJean Lawson, Ph.D., adjunct professor of exercise science at Oregon State University in Boring. "And you don't ever want to be without that again."

While the motivation to exercise comes from within, that doesn't mean you should sit in the lotus position and wait for it to strike. The tips below can help you muster up the motivation to start or stick with an exercise program.

Establish an inspiration space. Turn a small area in your kitchen, bedroom, or study into your personal shrine to fitness, suggests Marilyn Gansel, a certified personal trainer and the owner of Fitnessmatters in Stamford, Connecticut.

If you're frequently in the kitchen, for example, you could hang up a cork bulletin board and cover it with inspiring articles clipped from fitness magazines, news articles about ordinary women achieving extraordinary fitness goals, and motivational quotes. If you have a home gym in your basement, cover one entire wall with photos of women in motion—walking, dancing, lifting weights.

Reflect on your workout. If you exercise at home, invest in an inexpensive full-length mirror for your workout space. Watching your body get stronger and firmer will push you to continue. "Nothing motivates like results," says Williams-Evans.

Find a sweat buddy. Exercising with a friend, neighbor, or colleague makes it less likely that you'll blow off a scheduled workout, says Williams-Evans. "When you tell your workout buddy that you'll meet her at the gym, she shows up because she knows *you're* showing up, and vice versa. When it comes to exercise, many people break promises to themselves, but most won't let their friends down." Bonus: When the going gets tough (or dull), you'll have your own little cheering section.

As you progress in your program and begin to lift heavier and heavier weights, a buddy also doubles as a spotter. She can help you return the weight to its rack if your arms give out, or correct your technique if you're cheating a little without realizing it.

Buy motivation by the hour. Hire a personal trainer, even for two or three sessions, suggests Williams-Evans. If you're new to exercise, "a personal trainer can help you through the psychological discomfort of not knowing what you're doing, and the physical discomfort of using your body in new ways." If you've been exercising for a while, a trainer can boost your motivation by helping you devise a new workout or train for an event.

Think only celebrities can afford personal trainers? Think again. Depending on where you live, personal trainers may charge as little as $15 an hour, says Williams-Evans. Or you can hire a more expensive trainer and split the cost with a friend or two.

The trainer you choose should be certified by a national certification organization, such as the American Council on Exercise. She should also accommodate your schedule, have you fill out a personal health history to determine your needs

or limitations, and motivate with encouragement rather than bullying.

Ready, Set, Goal

Chances are, the last time you started a fitness program, you set a goal. To tone up. To slim down. To have more energy.

So how come you never quite made it?

It's not that setting goals doesn't work. "Research clearly shows that goal-setting not only helps people start a fitness program but also helps them stick with it," says Karla A. Kubitz, Ph.D., assistant professor of kinesiology at Towson University in Maryland.

The problem is that many of us set goals that are vague or unrealistic. Then, when we fail to meet them, our motivation to exercise bites the dust, says Dr. Kubitz.

It doesn't have to be that way. Here's how to set goals that work.

Include the how's, when's, and where's. "The more specific your goals, the more likely you are to meet them," says Bonnie Boyer, instructor in kinesiology at Pennsylvania State University in Schuylkill.

A vague goal such as "I want to get in shape" suddenly seems more doable when it's rewritten as, "For the next month, I will train with free weights for 1 hour after work on Mondays, Wednesdays, and Fridays."

Make timely goals. Give each goal a deadline, then use that date to keep yourself on track. But be realistic. You can expect to see results—feeling noticeably stronger and looking more toned—in a couple of months.

Set "now" and "later" goals. Break goals into two categories: long-term goals, which may take 6 months or more to achieve, and short-term goals, which you can accomplish in weeks or months. Meeting your short-term goals gives you a sense of pride and accomplishment that will keep you moving toward your long-term goals, says Dr. Kubitz.

Beware the fantasy goal. Make sure your goals are achievable, given your current level of fitness, your age, and your body type. "Setting extremely difficult or impossible goals is no better than not setting goals at all," says Dr. Kubitz.

Keep 'em coming. Devise new goals on a regular basis so your program and motivation stay fresh. "Goal-setting should be a dynamic process; keeping a journal of your goals and making a checklist is a good idea," says Boyer.

Shaking It Up

Think you'll scream if you watch any of the 57 workout videos in your collection one more time? Go mad if you do one more set of dumbbell flies? Go off the deep end if you swim one more lap in your local pool?

Sooner or later, boredom hits most exercisers. Exercise achievers have learned to recognize the danger signs—and deal with them—before boredom turns into burnout.

To turn your boredom back into enthusiasm, say experts, you need to reinject your program with fun, variety, and challenge. Here's how.

Determine (or reassess) your fitness personality. You stand a better chance of sticking to an exercise program for the long haul if you pick a workout that you actually enjoy, says Dr. Kubitz. Yet many people choose workouts that don't suit their temperaments.

To help you gain insight into your fitness personality, consider the following questions.

WOMAN TO WOMAN

She Gave Up Her Resistance to Resistance Training

From the time she was a little girl, Renee Bornstein hated to sweat. So she didn't—right up until she hit 41. Then a sudden crisis gave Renee, who runs a financial investigation company with her husband in Stamford, Connecticut, the incentive to start getting healthy. Here's her story.

As a kid, I hated physical activity. I was a chunky bookworm. So to me, team sports or being physically active was an absolute waste of time.

I lost the chunkiness in college, but not my dislike of exercise. I have vivid memories of high-school physical education class. We wore these ugly, light-blue gym uniforms, and our teacher was an absolute drill sergeant. It didn't matter if it was 150°F outside, we ran until we were dripping sweat. And I hate to sweat.

In college, I tried the aerobics thing—Jane Fonda had just hit it big. My sorority sisters were doing it, so I gave it a shot. As I said, I hate to sweat. So I quit that, too.

After I got married and had my kids, my weight problem returned with a vengeance. But still, I wouldn't exercise. I thought, "I have two babies. I don't have time."

What I did have was every excuse in the book.

The turning point came 2 years ago. I had three friends in their forties who were all diagnosed with breast cancer. I

Are you a people person? You're likely to enjoy exercise with a social component, such as swing dancing or a group Pilates class.

Are you the shy, quiet type? Solitary activities are likely to suit you. Consider cycling, inline skating, or swimming.

Do you enjoy playing "mental" games like chess? You may enjoy workouts that stress discipline and strategy, such as ballet, fencing, or the martial arts.

Play with neat new toys. Exercise balls, exercise tubes, rubber bands . . . your home gym or

was blown away. "This could happen to me," I thought. So I decided to get healthy. I committed myself to losing weight and exercising.

When I was a child, I loved to swim—it was probably the only athletic thing I did. So for my new exercise program, I joined a water-aerobics class. It sounded like fun: just a little splish-splashing in a pool.

Was I ever wrong. The instructor, who is now my personal trainer, worked me really hard. Still, I stuck with the class, and eventually, she asked me if I wanted to train with weights. And I thought, "Yuck . . . weights . . . sweating." But I'd made a commitment to get healthy, so I said yes. I also joined Weight Watchers and lost 15 pounds in a few months.

That was a year ago. Right now, I walk 5 days a week, take water-aerobics classes twice a week, and do resistance training once a week in an hour-long circuit, using free weights and a few machines.

It's the resistance training that has made the most difference in my body. When I started my program, my percentage of body fat was 42.9 percent. Now, it's down to 27.6 percent.

If anyone had told me 5 years ago that I'd be exercising regularly—and enjoying it—I'd have laughed out loud. Now, I know I'll be exercising for the rest of my life. I just wish I had started when I was a kid.

among them now and then. "The variety can help keep boredom from setting in," she says.

Make fitness eventful. Once you're in the swing of regular exercise, train for an event, suggests Dr. Kubitz. Train for a strenuous group hike or mountain-climbing expedition sponsored by a local outdoors club. If you cycle, enter a 20-mile ride with the local cycling group. The point isn't to win. It's to challenge your body and pump up your motivation.

Leaping the Fitness Hurdles

There are lots of reasons not to exercise, including the "I-just-don't-wannas." We shouldn't let any of them get in our way.

"Overcoming barriers to exercise is a lifelong struggle because there are always barriers," says Mary McElroy, Ph.D., professor in the department of kinesiology at Kansas State University in Manhattan, Kansas. "The key is to figure out ways to do that." These tips can help.

health club can become more like Romper Room when you play with the newest workout gear and gadgetry, says Williams-Evans. Who says you have to buy the stuff? Your health club may already have it. Or borrow it from a workout buddy.

Vary your routine. Once you've mastered the basics of your workout, learn new moves and routines, says Williams-Evans. Then vary among your repertoire each time you work out. There are nearly always several different exercises that will work each muscle, so switch

Determine your workout prime time. If you're a morning person, get in an energizing workout before starting your day. If you're a zombie before noon, exercise during your lunch hour or after work.

Put "too tired" to bed. Too exhausted to exercise? Probably not, says Dr. McElroy. If you've been sitting in an office or chauffeuring your kids around all day, it's probably your mind that's tired—and it needs the juice that a workout can provide. The next time you're "too tired" to exercise, says Dr. McElroy, "tell yourself, 'I realize I feel tired now. But once I start, I know I'll have more energy.'"

Dress for exercise success. Get dressed for your workout no matter how tired you feel or how sick to death you are of this whole exercise thing, says Dr. Lawson. Once you've slipped into your sweats and tied your sneaker laces, chances are, you'll actually feel like working out.

Schedule exercise appointments. Schedule your workouts into your day using a to-do list, a daily planner, or the scheduling software on your computer at work, just as you would a hair appointment or a meeting, says Gansel. Also, schedule your other obligations around your exercise session, rather than vice versa.

Make your workouts mom-friendly. If you have young children, either fit in a workout during your lunch hour or scout out a health club in your area that offers babysitting services, suggests Gansel.

Get back in the saddle. Many of us allow one missed workout—or several—to derail our fitness routines. Yet even the most dedicated exercisers occasionally get bored with their routines and fall into relapses. "It's important to acknowledge that relapses will occur from time to time," says Dr. McElroy. "Don't feel overly guilty about them. Just get back to working out."

Been AWOL from your program for longer than 2 weeks? Cut your routine in half and gradually work your way back, says Lisa Hoffman, an exercise physiologist, president of Solo Fitness, a personal training company based in New York City, and coauthor of *Better Than Ever: The 4-Week Workout Program for Women over 40*. A shorter workout will ease you back into your routine—and you'll avoid sore muscles, too.

Toning Up Your Awareness

If your workout is just another item to knock off your to-do list, it can be tough to muster up enthusiasm for your fitness routine, much less stick to it.

The solution: A mental technique called mindfulness, says Kylle Cooper, a certified fitness trainer at Miraval: Life in Balance, a spa/stress-reduction resort located in Catalina,

Arizona. Mindfulness—an intense awareness of what you're doing as you're doing it—can calm stress and make your workout a sort of moving meditation. But it also maximizes the benefits of a strength-training program by helping you to do the moves right, rather than fast.

"People who have worked out for years find that when they incorporate mindfulness into their workouts, they start to see better results," says Cooper. The tips below can help you get in mindful mode.

Come to your senses. Do you wear a stereo headset while you walk, or read on your exercise bike? Try tuning in to your workout, rather than tuning out, suggests Cooper.

At your next weight-training session, watch the way your left biceps—the muscle on the top of your upper arm—contracts as you lift your dumbbell and how it relaxes as you lower it. Notice how that feels. Concentrate on your breathing—your exhalation when you lift the weight, your inhalation when you lower it—and correct as necessary.

Slow down. When you rush through your workout, it's likely that your form is sloppy and you're not breathing properly, says Cooper. Such mindless workouts limit the benefits of your program and increase your risk of injury.

Lift and lower weights slowly, contracting your muscles hard as you do so. Breathe steadily and correctly. (No holding your breath.) Eventually, you may find that you can lift less weight and do fewer repetitions with equal or better results, says Cooper.

Index

Underscored page references indicate boxed text. **Boldface** references indicate illustrations.